Radiographic Positioning and Related Anatomy

Workbook and Laboratory Manual

VOLUME TWO

Chapters 14-24

Sixth Edition

Radiographic Positioning and Related Anatomy

Workbook and Laboratory Manual

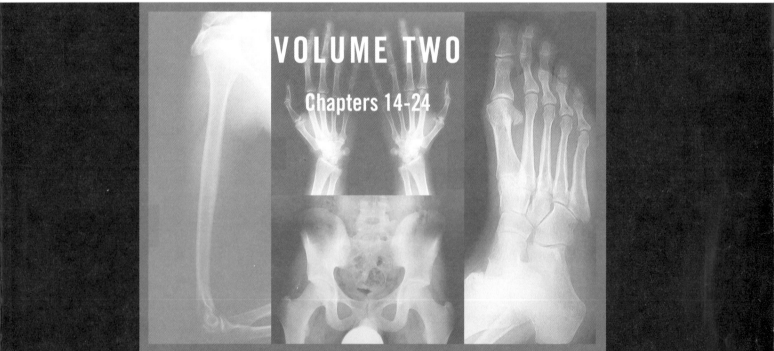

VOLUME TWO

Chapters 14-24

ELSEVIER
MOSBY

11830 Westline Industrial Drive
St. Louis, Missouri 63146

RADIOGRAPHIC POSITIONING AND
RELATED ANATOMY: WORKBOOK AND LABORATORY MANUAL,
6TH EDITION, VOLUME 2
Copyright © 2005, 2001, 1997 by Mosby, Inc.

NOTICE

Radiography is an ever-changing field. Standard safety precautions must be followed, but as new research and clinical experience broaden our knowledge, changes in treatment and drug therapy may become necessary or appropriate. Readers are advised to check the most current product information provided by the manufacturer of each drug to be administered to verify the recommended dose, the method and duration of administration, and contraindications. It is the responsibility of the licensed prescriber, relying on experience and knowledge of the patient, to determine dosages and the best treatment for each individual patient. Neither the publisher nor the author assumes any liability for any injury and/or damage to persons or property arising from this publication.

Executive Editor: Jeanne Wilke
Developmental Editor: Becky Swisher
Editorial Assistant: Christina Pryor
Publishing Services Manager: Pat Joiner
Senior Project Manager: Karen M. Rehwinkel
Senior Designer: Kathi Gosche

ISBN-13: 978-0-323-02505-8
ISBN-10: 0-323-02505-6

Printed in the United States of America

Last digit is the print number: 9   8   7   6   5   4   3   2

Acknowledgments

I am pleased to acknowledge and recognize those persons who have made significant contributions to the sixth edition of this student workbook and laboratory manual.

I first want to thank **John Lampignano,** who as co-author expanded the objectives and content of each chapter by submitting first drafts of additional questions for the new sections of the textbook. John is a very qualified and effective educator and has put a lot of effort and energy into this project. Thank you, John, for your excellent contributions.

I also thank **Jeanne Wilke, Karen Rehwinkel,** and **Rebecca Swisher** of the Mosby/Elsevier staff for their help and support in the preparation of this manuscript.

Last and most important, I want to thank my expanding family for their continued love, support, and encouragement and for bringing much joy and happiness into my life. I love each of you very much. Thanks **Mary Lou, Neil, Troy, Kim, Robyn, Hallie, Alexis, Ashton,** and **Jonathan**.

KLB

I would like to thank **Ken Bontrager** for his patience and mentorship in developing my skills as a writer. I've been honored to work with him over the past three editions. Ken has poured his heart and expertise into this text. Through his hard work and vision he has created a tremendous resource for students. **Mary Lou Bontrager** continues to provide the energy, technical support, and encouragement behind the scenes. Thank you, Mary Lou, for being there for both of us.

Ms. Rebecca Swisher, our associate editor, deserves praise for her dedication and vision in coordinating this project. She kept us on task and focused but always with a smile and a gentle word. Special thanks also to **Jeanne Wilke** for being a great editor and friend.

I would like to thank the diagnostic medical imaging faculty and clinical instructors at Gateway Community College who provide a shining example of excellence each and every day for our students and community. To my students—past, present, and future—you have made teaching a rewarding experience! Without your energy, laughter, and enthusiasm, teaching and writing this text would have been a burden rather than a joy. Finally, to my close friend, **Jerry Olson,** who taught me everything about radiography and many things about life—you have made my life richer and more worthwhile.

My family—**Deborah, Daniel,** and **Molly**—provide me with the greatest joy of all. I look at each of you and realize that I'm the luckiest person alive. Thank you for your love and support for the past 27 years. This book is dedicated to each of you.

JPL

Preface

The success of the first five editions of this workbook and laboratory manual and the accompanying textbook, along with the associated ancillary materials, is demonstrated by the many schools of radiologic technology throughout the United States, Canada, and other countries that have been using all or parts of these instructional media for more than 30 years.

New to This Edition

New illustrations and **expanded questions** have been added to reflect all the new content added to the sixth edition of *Textbook of Radiographic Positioning and Related Anatomy.* The use of visuals in these review exercises not only increases comprehension but also increases retention, because most individuals retain information most effectively through visual images.

The **detailed laboratory activities** have been updated, and the positioning question and answer exercises have been expanded, with less emphasis on rote memory recall. More **situational questions** involving **clinical applications** have been added. These questions aid in the understanding of positioning principles and of which anatomical structures are best demonstrated on which projections. The clinical situational questions added to each chapter require students to think through and understand how application of this positioning information relates to specific clinical examples.

Pathology questions have been expanded that will help students understand why they are performing specific exams and how exposure factors or positioning may be affected.

As in the textbook, entirely new sections added to the workbook include **digital radiography** and **surgical radiography.** The **bone densitometry** section has also been expanded, introductions to **nuclear medicine, PET radiation oncology, ultrasound imaging,** and **MRI** have also been revised and/or expanded.

How to Work with the Textbook and the Workbook and Laboratory Manuals

This sixth edition of the student workbook and laboratory manual is organized to be in complete agreement with the sixth edition of the *Textbook of Radiographic Positioning and Related Anatomy.* Each chapter in the textbook has a corresponding chapter in the workbook/manual to reinforce and supplement the information presented in the main text.

The most effective way to use this workbook/manual is for the student to complete the workbook chapter exercises immediately after reading and studying corresponding chapters in the textbook. To use both the student's and the instructor's time most effectively, this study should be done **before** the classroom presentation. The instructor can therefore spend more time in both the classroom and laboratory on problem areas and answering questions and less time on the fundamentals of anatomy and positioning, which students should already have learned.

Information for Faculty

ELECTRONIC ANCILLARIES (INSTRUCTORS ELECTRONIC RESOURCE CD)

These electronic resources are available on CD and consist of the following three components:

- **Computerized Test Bank (CTB) in Exam View**: This test bank features more than 2000 questions divided into the 24 chapters. It has been updated, expanded, and revised into more registry-level questions that can be used as final evaluation exams for each chapter. They can be used to produce paper-based exams, or they can be migrated into web-based course-authoring systems such as BlackBoard or WebCT, or test-authoring systems such as Respondus. Answer keys are provided for each examination.
- **Electronic Image Collection (EIC)**: Also available is an updated and expanded electronic image collection of images from all 24 chapters of the 6th edition of the textbook. These nonannotated images can be used by instructors for custom applications such as BlackBoard, Respondus, etc.
- **Electronic Instructional Presentation (EIP) in PowerPoint**: Now included is a new updated and epanded electronic image PowerPoint program that is fully coordinated with all 24 chapters of the 6th edition textbook and workbooks. These electronic images include text slides, some of which contain embedded anatomy and positioning images, resulting in a visually led instructional narrative. This can then be used as a complete chapter-by-chapter pre-programmed PowerPoint lecture guide. Sections from the more advanced chapters can also be used for in-service training or with post-graduate presentations.

Student Instructions

The following information will show you how to correctly use this workbook/laboratory manual and the accompanying textbook to help you master radiographic anatomy and positioning.

This course becomes the core of all your studies and your work as a radiologic technologist. **This is one course that you must master.** You cannot become a proficient technologist by marginally passing this course. Therefore please read these instructions carefully **before** beginning Chapter 1.

Objectives

Study the list of objectives carefully so that you will understand what you must know and be able to do after you complete each chapter.

Textbook and Workbook

Chapters 1 and **2** include a comprehensive introduction that prepares you for the remaining chapters of this positioning course. Your instructor may assign all or specific sections of these chapters at various times during your study of radiographic positioning and/or procedures.

Chapters 3-17 are specific positioning chapters that include the anatomy, positioning, and related procedures for all parts of the body.

Chapters 18-24 are more specialized procedures and modalities that are commonly studied later in a medical radiography program.

Learning Exercises

These exercises are the focal point of this workbook/laboratory manual. Using them correctly will help you learn and remember the important information presented in each chapter of the textbook. To maximize the benefits from each exercise, **follow the correct six-step order of activities** as outlined below.

ANATOMY ACTIVITIES

Step 1. (Textbook): Carefully read and learn the **radiographic anatomy** section of each of these chapters. Include the anatomic reviews on labeled radiographs provided in the textbook. Pay particular attention to those items in **bold type** and to the **summary review boxes,** where provided.

Step 2. (Workbook, Part I): Complete Part I of the review exercises on **radiographic anatomy.** Do **not** look up the answers in the textbook or look at the answer sheet until you have answered as many of the questions as you can. Then refer to the textbook and/or the answer sheet and correct or complete those questions you missed. Reread those sections of the textbook in which you could not answer questions. Textbook page numbers are provided next to each review exercise in this workbook.

POSITIONING ACTIVITIES

Step 3. (Textbook): Carefully read and study Part II on all of the parts on **radiographic positioning.** Note the general **positioning considerations, alternate modalities,** and **pathologic indications** for each chapter. Information from these sections will be seen on workbook review exercises, self-tests, and chapter evaluations. This is followed by the specific positioning pages, which include **pathology demonstrated, technical factors,** and the **dose ranges** of skin, midline, and specific organ doses, where provided. Pay particular attention to dose comparisons between different techniques, or anteroposterior (AP) versus posteroanterior (PA) projections. Learn the **specific positioning steps,** the **central ray location and angle,** and the four-part **radiographic criteria** for each projection or position.

Part II: Radiographic Positioning

REVIEW EXERCISE C: Contrast Media, Fluoroscopy, and Pathologic Indications and Contraindications for Upper Gastrointestinal Studies (see textbook pp. 456-470)

1. True/False: With the use of digital fluoroscopy, the number of postfluoroscopy radiographs ordered has greatly diminished.

2. What is the most common form of positive contrast medium used for studies of the gastrointestinal system?

   _____

3. Another term for a negative contrast medium is _____

4. What substance is most commonly ingested to produce carbon dioxide gas as a negative contrast medium for

   gastrointestinal studies? _____

5. Is a mixture of barium sulfate a suspension or a solution? _____

6. True/False: Barium sulfate never dissolves in water.

7. True/False: Certain salts of barium are poisonous to humans, so barium contrast studies require a pure sulfate salt of barium for human consumption during GI studies.

8. What is the ratio of water to barium for a thin mixture of barium sulfate? _____

9. What is the chemical symbol for barium sulfate? _____

10. When is the use of barium sulfate contraindicated? _____

11. What patient condition would prevent the use of a water-soluble contrast media for an upper GI?

    _____

12. What is the major advantage for using a double-contrast media technique for esophagrams and upper GIs?

    _____.

13. The speed with which barium sulfate passes through the GI tract is called gastric _____.

14. What is the purpose of the gas with a double-contrast media technique?

    _____

15. Conventional image intensification:

    A. The photospot or cine images, such as recorded on a 105-mm film, are taken from the _____ (**input** or **output**) side of the image intensifier.

    B. Conventional spot film images on 18×24 cm (8×10 in) cassettes are recorded from the

       _____ (**input** or **output**) side of the image intensifier.

    C. Which of the images described above is the brighter image—A or B? _____

    D. How many times brighter is the fluoroscopic image when enhanced or brightened by the image intensifier? _____

16. What device (found beneath the radiographic table when correctly positioned) greatly reduces exposure to the technologist from the fluoroscopic x-ray tube?

    A. Lead skirt   B. Lead drape   C. Bucky slot shield   D. Fluoroscopy tube shield

17. How is the device referred to in question 16 activated or placed in its correct position for fluoroscopy?

    _____

18. What is the major benefit of using a compression paddle during an upper GI study?

    A. Reduces exposure to the patient   C. Reduces exposure to arms and hands of radiologist

    B. Reduces exposure to the eyes of radiologist   D. Reduces exposure to the torso of radiologist

19. During an upper GI fluoroscopy procedure, if the technologist stands directly beside the radiologist next to the patient's head and shoulders (see textbook, p. 68), zone C in Fig. 2-53, how much radiation would the technologist receive to the lead apron at waist level during each fluoroscopic exam if the radiologist averaged 5 minutes of fluoroscopy exposure per patient? (HINT: determine exposure dose range in mR/min in zone C and multiply by 5 minutes.)

    _____

20. Where is the best place for the technologist to stand during an upper GI procedure, and how much exposure would he or she receive in that position with 5 minutes of fluoroscopy?

    _____

21. List the three cardinal principles of radiation protection:

    A. _____

    B. _____

    C. _____

22. Which one of the three cardinal principles is most effective in reducing exposure to the technologist during a fluoroscopic procedure?

    _____

23. List the six advantages or unique features and capabilities of digital fluoroscopy over conventional fluoroscopic recording systems:

    A. _____

    B. _____

    C. _____

    D. _____

    E. _____

    F. _____

24. What is another term that describes intermittent "road mapping" when used in digital fluoroscopy?

    _____

25. Match the following definitions or descriptions to the correct pathologic indication for the esophagram:

    _____ A. Difficulty in swallowing

    _____ B. Replacement of normal squamous epithelium with columnar epithelium

    _____ C. May lead to esophagitis

    _____ D. May be secondary to cirrhosis of the liver

    _____ E. Large outpouching of the esophagus

    _____ F. Also called *cardiospasm*

    _____ G. Most common form is adenocarcinoma

    1. Achalasia

    2. Zenker's diverticulum

    3. Esophageal varices

    4. Carcinoma of esophagus

    5. Barrett's esophagus

    6. GERD

    7. Dysphagia

26. Match the following definitions or descriptions to the correct pathologic indication for the upper GI series:

    _____ A. Blood in vomit

    _____ B. Inflammation of lining of stomach

    _____ C. Blind outpouching of the mucosal wall

    _____ D. Undigested material trapped in stomach

    _____ E. Synonymous with gastric or duodenal ulcer

    _____ F. Portion of stomach protruding through diaphragmatic opening

    _____ G. Only 5% of ulcers lead to this condition

    _____ H. Double-contrast upper GI is the gold standard for diagnosing this condition

    1. Hiatal hernia

    2. Gastric carcinoma

    3. Bezoar

    4. Hematemesis

    5. Gastritis

    6. Perforating ulcer

    7. Peptic ulcer

    8. Diverticula

27. Match the following pathologic conditions or diseases to the correct radiographic appearance:

    _____ A. Its presence indicates a possible sliding hiatal hernia

    _____ B. Speckled appearance of gastric mucosa

    _____ C. "Wormlike" appearance of esophagus

    _____ D. Stricture of esophagus

    _____ E. Gastric bubble above diaphragm

    _____ F. Irregular filling defect within stomach

    _____ G. Enlarged recess in proximal esophagus

    _____ H. "Lucent-halo" sign during upper GI

    1. Ulcers

    2. Hiatal hernia

    3. Achalasia

    4. Zenker's diverticulum

    5. Schatzke's ring

    6. Gastritis

    7. Esophageal varices

    8. Gastric carcinoma

28. Which procedure is often performed to detect early signs of GERD? _____

29. Which specific structure of the gastrointestinal system is affected by HPS?

_____

30. Which imaging modality is most effective in diagnosing HPS while reducing dose to the patient?

_____

REVIEW EXERCISE D: Patient Preparation and Positioning for Esophagram and Upper Gastrointestinal Study (see textbook pp. 471-483)

1. What does the acronym NPO stand for, and what does it mean? _____

2. True/False: The patient must be NPO 4 to 6 hours before an esophagram.

3. True/False: The esophagram usually begins with fluoroscopy with the patient in the erect position.

4. What materials may be used for swallowing to aid in the diagnosis of radiolucent foreign bodies in the esophagus?

_____

5. List the four tests that may be performed to detect signs of GERD (esophageal reflux):

   A. _____   C. _____

   B. _____   D. _____

6. A breathing technique in which the patient takes in a deep breath and bears down is called the

_____ .

7. What position is the patient usually placed in during the water test? _____

8. Which region of the GI tract is better visualized when the radiologist uses a compression paddle during an

   esophagram? _____

9. What type of contrast media should be used if the patient has a history of bowel perforation?

_____ .

10. What is the minimum amount of time that the patient should be NPO before an upper GI? _____ .

11. Why should cigarette and gum chewing be restricted before an upper GI?

_____ .

12. Why should the technologist review the patient's chart before the beginning of an upper GI?
    A. Identify any known allergies   C. Look for pertinent clinical history
    B. Ensure that the proper study has been ordered   D. All of the above

13. In which hand does the patient usually hold the barium cup during the start of an upper GI? _____

14. List the suggested dosages of barium sulfate during an upper GI for each of the following pediatric age groups:

   Newborn to 1 year: _____

   1 to 3 years: _____

   3 to 10 years: _____

   Over 10 years: _____

15. What is the name of the special adapter attached to a syringe to deliver contrast media through a nasogastric tube?

   _____

16. Which one of the following imaging modalities is an alternative to an esophagram in detecting esophageal varices?
   A. Nuclear medicine   C. Sonography
   B. Computed tomography   D. None of the above

17. Gastric emptying studies are performed using:
   A. Intraesophageal sonography   C. Magnetic resonance
   B. Radionuclides   D. Computed tomography

18. Why is the RAO preferred over the LAO for an esophagram?

   _____

19. How much rotation of the body should be used for the RAO projection of the esophagus? _____

20. Which optional position should be performed to demonstrate the upper esophagus located between the shoulders?

   _____

21. Which aspect of the GI tract is best demonstrated with an RAO position during an upper GI?
   A. Fundus of stomach   C. Body of stomach
   B. Pylorus of stomach and C-loop   D. Fourth (ascending) portion of duodenum

22. How much rotation of the body should be used for the RAO position during an upper GI on a sthenic patient?
   A. 30° to 35°   C. 40° to 70°
   B. 15° to 20°   D. 10° to 15°

23. What is the average kV range for an esophagram and upper GI when using barium sulfate (without double-contrast

   study)? _____

24. Which aspect of the upper GI tract will be filled with barium in the PA projection (prone position)?

   _____

25. What is the purpose of the PA axial projection for the hypersthenic patient during an upper GI?

   _____

26. What CR angle is used for the PA axial projection?

    A. 10° to 15° caudad   C. 35° to 45° cephalad

    B. 20° to 25° cephalad   D. 60° to 70° cephalad

27. Which projection taken during an upper GI will best demonstrate the retrogastric space?

    A. RAO   C. LPO

    B. Lateral   D. PA

28. A double-contrast upper GI requires a slightly _____ (**higher** or **lower**) kV compared with a single-contrast medium study.

29. The female gonadal dose range for a well-collimated RAO projection of the upper GI procedure is:

    A. 10 to 15 mrad   C. 200 to 500 mrad

    B. 50 to 100 mrad   D. 600 to 1000 mrad

30. The upper GI series usually begins with the table and patient in the _____ position.

31. The five most common basic or routine projections for an upper GI series are (not counting a possible AP scout image):

    A. _____   C. _____   E. _____

    B. _____   D. _____

32. The three most common basic or routine projections for an esophagram are:

    A. _____   B. _____   C. _____

33. The major parts of the stomach on an average patient are usually confined to which abdominal quadrant?

    _____

34. Most of the duodenum is usually found to the _____ (**right** or **left**) of the midline on an average patient.

35. True/False: Respiration should be suspended during inspiration for upper GI radiographic projections.

REVIEW EXERCISE E: Problem Solving for Technical and Positioning Errors (see textbook pp. 463-483)

1. **Situation:** A radiograph of an RAO projection taken during an esophagram demonstrates incomplete filling of the esophagus with barium. What can the technologist do to ensure better filling of the esophagus during the repeat exposure?

_____

_____

2. **Situation:** A series of radiographs taken during an upper GI reveal that the stomach mucosa is not well visualized. The following factors were used during this positioning routine: high-speed screens, Bucky, 40-inch (102-cm) SID, 80 kV, 30 mAs, and 300 ml of barium sulfate ingested during the procedure. Which exposure factor should be changed to produce a more diagnostic study?

    _____

    _____

3. **Situation:** A radiograph taken during an upper GI reveals that the anatomic side marker is missing. The technologist is unsure whether it is a recumbent AP or PA projection. The fundus of the stomach is filled with barium. Which position does this radiograph represent?

    _____

    _____

4. **Situation:** A radiograph of an RAO projection taken during an upper GI reveals that the duodenal bulb is not well demonstrated and not profiled. The RAO was a 45° oblique performed on a hypersthenic-type patient. What positioning modification needs to be made to produce a better image of the duodenal bulb?

    _____

    _____

5. **Situation:** A radiograph of an upper GI was taken, but the student technologist is unsure of the position. The radiograph demonstrates that the fundus is filled with barium, but the duodenal bulb is air-filled and seen in profile. Which position does this radiograph represent?

    _____

    _____

6. **Situation:** A patient with a clinical history of hiatal hernia comes to the radiology department. Which procedure should be performed on this patient to rule out this condition?

    _____

7. **Situation:** A patient with a possible lacerated duodenum enters the emergency room. The ER physician orders an upper GI to determine the extent of the injury. What type of contrast media should be used for this examination?

    _____

    _____

8. **Situation:** A patient with a fish bone stuck in his esophagus enters the emergency room. What modification to a standard esophagram may be needed to locate the foreign body?

    _____

    _____

9. **Situation:** An upper GI is being performed on a thin, asthenic-type patient. Because of room scheduling conflicts, this patient was brought into your room for the overhead follow-up images following fluoroscopy. Where would you center the CR and the 11 × 14 inch (30 × 35 cm) image receptor to ensure that you included the stomach and duodenal regions?

_____

_____

10. **Situation:** A patient with a clinical history of a possible bezoar comes to the radiology department. What is a bezoar, and what radiographic study should be performed to demonstrate this condition?

_____

_____

11. **Situation:** A radiograph of an RAO position taken during an esophagram reveals that the esophagus is superimposed over the vertebral column. What positioning error led to this radiographic outcome? What must be altered to eliminate this problem during the repeat exposure?

_____

_____

12. **Situation:** A PA projection taken during an upper GI series performed on an infant reveals that the body and pylorus of the stomach are superimposed. What modification needs to be employed during the repeat exposure to separate these two regions?

_____

_____

13. **Situation:** A patient comes to radiology with a clinical history of possible gastric diverticulum in the posterior aspect of the fundus. Which projection taken during the upper GI series will best demonstrate this defect?

_____

_____

14. **Situation:** A patient comes to radiology with a clinical history of Barrett's esophagus. In addition to an esophagram, what other imaging modality is ideal in demonstrating this condition?

_____

_____

15. **Situation:** A patient has a clinical history of hemochromatosis. Which imaging modality is most effective in diagnosing this condition?

_____

_____

Part III: Laboratory Exercises (see textbook pp. 475-483)

You must gain experience in positioning each part of the esophagram and upper GI procedures before performing the following exams on actual patients. You can get experience in positioning and radiographic evaluation of these projections by performing exercises using radiographic phantoms and practicing on other students (although you will not be taking actual exposures).

LABORATORY EXERCISE A: Radiographic Evaluation

1. Evaluate and critique the radiographs produced during the previous experiments, additional radiographs of esophagrams and upper GI procedures provided by your instructor, or both. Evaluate each position for the following points (check off when completed):

   _____ Evaluate the completeness of the study. (Are all the pertinent anatomic structures included on the radiograph?)

   _____ Evaluate for positioning or centering errors (e.g., rotation, off centering).

   _____ Evaluate for correct exposure factors and possible motion. (Are the density and contrast of the images acceptable?)

   _____ Determine whether markers and an acceptable degree of collimation and/or area shielding are visible on the images.

LABORATORY EXERCISE B: Physical Positioning

On another person, simulate performing all basic and special projections of the upper GI as follows. Include the six steps listed below and described in the textbook. (Check off each when completed satisfactorily.)

Step 1. Appropriate size and type of image receptor holder with correct markers
Step 2. Correct CR placement and centering of part to CR and/or image receptor
Step 3. Accurate collimation
Step 4. Area shielding of patient where advisable
Step 5. Use of proper immobilizing devices when needed
Step 6. Approximate correct exposure factors, breathing instructions where applicable, and "making" exposure

PROJECTIONS	STEP 1	STEP 2	STEP 3	STEP 4	STEP 5	STEP 6
• RAO esophagram	____	____	____	____	____	____
• Left lateral esophagram	____	____	____	____	____	____
• AP (PA) esophagram	____	____	____	____	____	____
• LAO esophagram	____	____	____	____	____	____
• Soft tissue lateral esophagram	____	____	____	____	____	____
• RAO upper GI	____	____	____	____	____	____
• PA upper GI	____	____	____	____	____	____
• Right lateral upper GI	____	____	____	____	____	____
• LPO upper GI	____	____	____	____	____	____
• AP upper GI	____	____	____	____	____	____

Answers to Review Exercises

Review Exercise A: Radiographic Anatomy of the Upper Gastrointestinal System

1. A. Mouth
   B. Pharynx
   C. Esophagus
   D. Stomach
   E. Small intestine
   F. Large intestine
   G. Anus
2. A. Salivary glands
   B. Pancreas
   C. Liver
   D. Gallbladder
3. A. Intake and digestion of food
   B. Absorption of digested food particles
   C. Elimination of solid waste products
4. Esophagram or barium swallow
5. Upper gastrointestinal (UGI) series, or upper GI
6. A. Parotid
   B. Sublingual
   C. Submandibular
7. Deglutition
8. A. Nasopharynx
   B. Oropharynx
   C. Laryngopharynx
9. A. Aortic arch
   B. Left primary bronchus
10. A. Esophagus
    B. Inferior vena cava
    C. Aorta
11. Duodenal bulb or cap
12. Duodenojejunal flexure (suspensory ligament or ligament of Trietz)
13. Retroperitoneal (or "behind peritoneum")
14. A. Tongue
    B. Oral cavity (mouth)
    C. Hard palate
    D. Soft palate
    E. Uvula
    F. Nasopharynx
    G. Oropharynx
    H. Epiglottis
    I. Laryngopharynx
    J. Larynx
    K. Esophagus
    L. Trachea
15. A. Erect
    B. Prone
    C. Supine
16. False (inferiorly and anteriorly)
17. A. Fundus
    B. Greater curvature
    C. Body
    D. Gastric canal

E. Pyloric portion
F. Pyloric orifice (or just pylorus)
G. Angular notch (incisura angularis)
H. Lesser curvature
I. Esophagogastric junction (cardiac orifice)
J. Cardiac antrum
K. Cardiac notch (incisura cardiaca)
18. A. Fundus (labeled A on Fig. 14-3)
    B. Body or corpus (labeled C)
    C. Pyloric (labeled E)
19. Pyloric antrum and pyloric canal
20. Rugae
21. A. Pylorus (pyloric sphincter)
    B. Bulb or cap of duodenum
    C. First (superior) portion of duodenum
    D. Second (descending) portion of duodenum
    E. Third (horizontal) portion of duodenum
    F. Fourth (ascending) portion of duodenum
    G. Head of pancreas
    H. Suspensory ligament of duodenum or ligament of Treitz
22. A. Head of pancreas
    B. C-loop of duodenum
23. A. Distal esophagus
    B. Area of esophagogastric junction
    C. Lesser curve of stomach
    D. Angular notch (incisura angularis)
    E. Pyloric region of stomach
    F. Pyloric valve or sphincter
    G. Duodenal bulb
    H. Second descending portion of duodenum
    I. Body of stomach
    J. Greater curvature of stomach
    K. Gastric folds or rugae of stomach
    L. Fundus of stomach

Review Exercise B: Mechanical and Chemical Digestion and Body Habitus

1. True
2. A. Pharynx
3. Chyme
4. Rhythmic segmentation
5. A. Carbohydrates
   B. Proteins
   C. Lipids (fats)
6. Enzymes
7. A. Simple sugars
   B. Fatty acids and glycerol
   C. Amino acids
8. Bile
9. A. Small intestine
   B. Stomach
10. Bile

11. Carbohydrates
12. Large intestine
13. Mechanical
14. Chyme
15. A. Hypersthenic
16. C. Hyposthenic/asthenic
17. 1 to 2 inches (2.5 to 5 cm)
18. A. Stomach
    B. Gallbladder
19. Inferior, because of its proximity to the diaphragm
20. 1. A, B
    2. B
    3. B, C
    4. C, D
    5. C, E

Review Exercise C: Contrast Media, Fluoroscopy, and Pathologic Indications and Contraindications for Upper Gastrointestinal Studies

1. True
2. Barium sulfate
3. Radiolucent contrast medium
4. Calcium carbonate
5. Suspension
6. True
7. True
8. One part water to one part barium sulfate (1:1 ratio)
9. $BaSO_4$
10. When the mixture may escape into the peritoneal cavity (p. 458)
11. Sensitivity to iodine
12. Better coating and visibility of the mucosa. Polyps, diverticula, and ulcers are better demonstrated.
13. Motility
14. It forces the barium sulfate against the mucosa for better coating.
15. A. Output
    B. Input
    C. A. Photospot or cine images are brighter
    D. 1000 to 6000 times
16. C. Bucky slot shield
17. By moving the Bucky all the way to the end of the table
18. C. Reduces exposure to arms and hands of radiologist
19. $1.7 - 3.3 \times 5 = 8.5 - 16.5$ mRad
20. Away from the patient and table and/or behind the radiologist (zone F). Would receive less than 2.0 mrad ($0.4 \times 5 = 2.0$ mrad).
21. A. Time
    B. Distance
    C. Shielding

14

22. Distance
23. A. No cassettes required
    B. Optional postfluoroscopy over-head images
    C. Multiple frame formatting and multiple original IRs
    D. Cine loop capability
    E. Image enhancement and manip-ulation (by computers)
    F. Reduced patient exposure (by as much as 30% to 50%)
24. "Frame hold" capability of specific fluoroscopy images
25. A. 7
    B. 5
    C. 6
    D. 3
    E. 2
    F. 1
    G. 4
26. A. 4
    B. 5
    C. 8
    D. 3
    E. 7
    F. 1
    G. 6
    H. 2
27. A. 5
    B. 6
    C. 7
    D. 3
    E. 2
    F. 8
    G. 4
    H. 1
28. Endoscopy
29. Antral muscle at the orifice of the pylorus
30. Ultrasound (sonography)

Review Exercise D: Patient Preparation and Positioning for Esophagram and Upper Gastrointestinal Study

1. Literally stands for *non per os,* a Latin phrase meaning "nothing by mouth" (p. 471)
2. False (8 hours NPO for upper GI but not for an esophagram)
3. True
4. Barium-soaked cotton balls, barium pills, or marshmallows followed by thin barium
5. A. Breathing exercises
   B. Water test
   C. Compression technique
   D. Toe-touch maneuver
6. Valsalva maneuver
7. LPO
8. Esophagogastric junction

9. Oral, water-soluble iodinated con-trast media
10. 8 hours
11. Both activities tend to increase gas-tric secretions.
12. D. All of the above
13. Left hand
14. Newborn to 1 year: 2 to 4 ounces
    1 to 3 years: 4 to 6 ounces
    3 to 10 years: 6 to 12 ounces
    Over 10 years: 12 to 16 ounces
15. Christmas tree or tapered adapter
16. C. Sonography
17. B. Radionuclides
18. Places the esophagus between the vertebral column and heart
19. 35° to 40°
20. Optional swimmer's lateral
21. B. Pylorus of stomach and C-loop
22. C. 40° to 70°
23. 100 to 125 kV
24. Body and pylorus of stomach and duodenal bulb
25. To prevent superimposition of the pylorus over the duodenal bulb, and to better visualize the lesser and greater curvatures of the stomach
26. C. 35° to 45° cephalad
27. B. Lateral
28. Lower
29. A. 10 to 15 mrad
30. Upright (erect)
31. A. RAO
    B. PA
    C. Right lateral
    D. LPO
    E. AP
32. A. RAO
    B. Left lateral
    C. AP
33. Left upper quadrant (LUQ)
34. Right
35. False (expiration)

Review Exercise E: Problem Solving for Technical and Positioning Errors

1. When using thin barium, have the patient drink continuously during the exposure. With thick barium, have the patient hold two or three spoonfuls in the mouth and make the exposure immediately after swallowing.
2. When using barium sulfate as a con-trast media, 110 to 125 kV should be used to ensure proper penetra-tion of the contrast-filled stomach and to visualize the mucosa. 80 to 100 kV would be adequate for a double-contrast study.

3. AP. Since the fundus is more poste-rior than the body or pylorus, it will fill with barium when the patient is in a supine (AP) position.
4. With a hypersthenic patient, more rotation (up to 70°) may be required to better profile the duode-nal bulb. (NOTE: The radiologist under fluoroscopic guidance will fre-quently move the patient obliquely as needed for the overhead oblique to best profile the duodenal region. Observe the degree of rotation of the body required to profile the stomach during fluoroscopy.)
5. The LPO position (recumbent) will produce an image in which the fun-dus and body are filled with barium but the duodenal bulb is air-filled.
6. Upper GI series
7. An oral, water-soluble contrast media should be used for an upper GI when ruptured viscus or bowel is suspected (not barium sulfate, which is not water-soluble).
8. With radiolucent foreign bodies in the esophagus, shredded cotton soaked in barium sulfate may be used to help locate it. Marshmallows with barium or a bar-ium capsule may also be used.
9. Would center lower than usual, to the mid-L3 to L4 region or about 1½ to 2 inches (4 to 5 cm) above the level of the iliac crest
10. A mass of undigested material that gets trapped in the stomach; a rare condition that can be diagnosed with an upper GI study.
11. Underrotation of the body into the RAO position led to the esophagus being superimposed over the ver-tebral column. An increase in rota-tion of the body during the repeat exposure will separate the esopha-gus from the spine.
12. Angle the CR 20° to 25° cephalad to open up the body and pylorus of the stomach.
13. The lateral position will best demon-strate a gastric diverticulum located in the posterior region of the stomach.
14. Nuclear medicine is an effective modality in detecting Barrett's esophagus.
15. Hemochromatosis is a condition of abnormal iron deposits in the liver parenchyma. Magnetic resonance imaging (MRI) is an effective imag-ing modality in diagnosing this condition.

SELF-TEST

My Score = _____ %

Directions: This self-test should be taken only after completing all of the readings, review exercises, and laboratory activities. The purpose of this test is not only to provide a good learning exercise but also to serve as a good indicator of what your final evaluation exam will be. It is strongly suggested that if you do not get at least a 90% to 95% grade on this self-test, you review those areas where you missed questions before going to your instructor for the final evaluation exam for this chapter. (There are 87 questions or blanks—each is worth 1.5 points.)

1. Which one of the following is **not** a function of the gastrointestinal system?

    A. Intake and digestion of food   C. Production of hormones

    B. Absorption of nutrients   D. Elimination of waste products

2. Which one of the following is **not** a salivary gland?

    A. Parotid   C. Pineal

    B. Sublingual   D. Submandibular

3. What is another term for an esophagram? _____

4. What is the name of the condition that results from a viral infection of the parotid gland? _____

5. The act of chewing is termed:

    A. Mastication   C. Aspiration

    B. Deglutition   D. Peristalsis

6. Which structure in the pharynx prevents aspiration of food and fluid into the larynx?

    A. Uvula   C. Soft palate

    B. Epiglottis   D. Laryngopharynx

7. The esophagus extends from C5-6 to:

    A. T9   C. T10

    B. L1   D. T11

8. Which one of the following structures does not pass through the diaphragm?

    A. Trachea   C. Aorta

    B. Esophagus   D. Inferior vena cava

9. Wavelike involuntary contractions that help propel food down the esophagus are called _____ .

10. The Greek term *gaster,* or *gastro,* means _____ .

11. Which one of the following aspects of the stomach is defined as an indentation between the body and pylorus?

    A. Cardiac antrum   C. Incisura cardiaca

    B. Pyloric antrum   D. Incisura angularis

12. Which aspect of the stomach will fill with air when the patient is prone?

    A. Fundus   C. Duodenal bulb

    B. Body   D. Pylorus

13. True/False: The numerous mucosal folds found in the small bowel are called *rugae*.

14. True/False: The lateral margin of the stomach is called the *lesser curvature*.

15. Which aspect of the stomach will barium gravitate to when the patient is in the supine position? _____

16. Which two structures create the "romance of the abdomen"? _____

17. Match each of the following aspects of the upper gastrointestinal system with the correct definition.

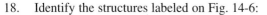

_____ 1. Pyloric orifice	A. Middle aspect of stomach
_____ 2. Cardiac notch	B. Horizontal portion of duodenum
_____ 3. Fundus	C. Rugae
_____ 4. Fourth portion of duodenum	D. Opening between esophagus and stomach
_____ 5. Gastric folds	E. Opening leaving the stomach
_____ 6. Body	F. Found along superior aspect of fundus
_____ 7. Esophagogastric junction	G. Indentation found along lesser curvature
_____ 8. Angular notch	H. Ascending portion of duodenum
_____ 9. Third portion of duodenum	I. Most posterior aspect of stomach

18. Identify the structures labeled on Fig. 14-6:

A. _____

B. _____

C. _____

D. _____

E. _____

F. _____

G. _____

H. _____

I. _____

J. _____

K. _____

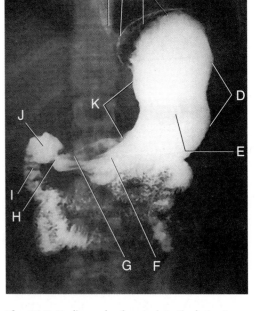

Fig. 14-6. Radiograph of gastrointestinal structures, demonstrating body position.

19. A. Which body position does Fig. 14-6 represent? _____

    B. How could you determine this? _____

20.   Which body position does Fig. 14-7 represent? _____

21.   A.   Which body position does Fig. 14-8 represent? _____

      B.   How could you determine this? _____

22.   A.   Fig. 14-9 represents a(n) _____ (**anterior** or **posterior**) oblique position.

      B.   How could you determine this? _____

      C.   Which specific oblique position does Fig. 14-10 represent? _____

      D.   How could you determine this? _____

23.   Which term describes food once it enters the stomach and is mixed with gastric fluids? _____

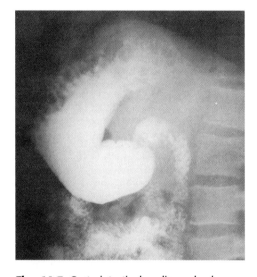

Fig. 14-7. Gastrointestinal radiograph demonstrating body position.

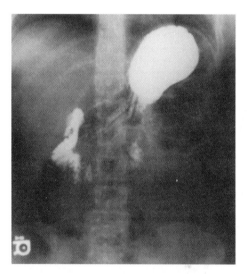

Fig. 14-8. Gastrointestinal radiograph demonstrating body position.

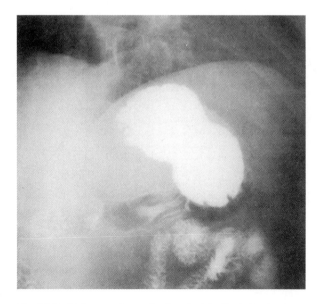

Fig. 14-9. Oblique radiograph of gastrointestinal structures.

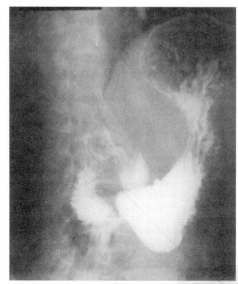

Fig. 14-10. Oblique radiograph of gastrointestinal structures.

14

24. Which one of the following nutrients is not digested?

    A. Vitamins   C. Carbohydrates

    B. Lipids   D. Proteins

25. The churning or mixing activity of chyme in the small intestine is called:

    A. Peristalsis   C. Rhythmic segmentation

    B. Deglutition   D. Digestion

26. A _____ or _____ type of body habitus will usually have a

    low and vertical stomach with the pyloric portion of the stomach at the level of _____ .

27. A high and transverse stomach indicates a _____ body type with the pyloric portion at

    the level of _____ .

28. What is the most common radiopaque contrast media used in the gastrointestinal system?

    _____

29. What type of radiolucent contrast medium is most commonly used for double-contrast gastrointestinal studies?

    _____

30. A. What is the ratio of barium to water for a thick mixture of barium sulfate? _____

    B. What is the ratio for a thin barium mixture? _____

31. When should a water-soluble contrast media be used during an upper GI rather than barium sulfate?

    _____

32. Which one of the following conditions may prevent the use of water-soluble contrast agents for a geriatric patient?

    A. Bowel obstruction   C. Dehydration

    B. Chronic aspiration   D. Perforated ulcer

33. True/False: Water-soluble contrast agents pass through the gastrointestinal tract faster than barium sulfate.

34. Cinefluorography cameras record the image from the _____ (**input** or **output**) side of the image intensifier.

35. Image-intensified fluoroscopy is brighter than older conventional fluoroscopy without intensifiers.

    A. 100 times   C. 1000 to 6000 times

    B. 10 times   D. 10,000 to 60,000 times

36. True/False: Digital fluoroscopy does not require the use of image receptor cassettes.

37. Digital fluoroscopy leads to _____ (**higher** or **lower**) patient dose as compared with conventional fluoroscopy.

38. Which of the cardinal principles of radiation protection is most effective in reducing exposure to the technologist

    during fluoroscopy? _____

39. Protective aprons of _____ lead equivalency must be worn during fluoroscopy?

    A. 1.0 mm Pb/Eq   C. 0.25 mm Pb/Eq

    B. 0.50 mm Pb/Eq   D. 0.15 mm Pb/Eq

40. A large outpouching of the upper esophagus is termed:

    A. Zenker's diverticulum   C. Barrett's esophagus

    B. Achalasia   D. Esophageal varices

41. Which one of the following is the older term for GERD?

    A. Esophageal reflux   C. Esophageal varices

    B. Barrett's esophagus   D. Zenker's diverticulum

42. What criterion is used with ultrasound in determining whether a patient has HPS?

    A. Abnormally long pylorus   C. Presence of air-fluid level in the duodenum

    B. Absence of rugae   D. Antral muscle thickness exceeding 4 mm

43. Other than the esophagram, what other imaging modality is performed to diagnose Barrett's esophagus?

    A. Computed tomography   C. Magnetic resonance

    B. Nuclear medicine   D. Sonography

44. A phytobezoar is:

    A. An outpouching of the mucosal wall   C. A rare tumor

    B. Trapped mass of hair in the stomach   D. Trapped vegetable fiber in the stomach

45. What is the reason that the patient may be asked to swallow a mouthful of water drawn through a straw during an esophagram?

    _____

46. How much rotation of the body should be used for the RAO esophagram projection? _____

47. Why is an RAO position preferred rather than an LAO during an esophagram?

    _____

48. Why is the AP projection of the esophagus not a preferred projection for the esophagram series?

    _____

49. What can be added to the barium sulfate and swallowed to detect a radiolucent foreign body lodged in the esophagus?

    _____

50. Which upper GI position will best demonstrate a possible gastric diverticulum in the posterior wall of the fundus of

    the stomach? _____

14

51. **Situation:** An upper GI series is performed on an asthenic patient. A radiograph of the RAO position reveals that the duodenal bulb and C loop are not in profile. The technologist rotated the patient 50 degrees. What modification of the position is required during the repeat exposure?

_____

52. A radiograph taken during a double-contrast upper GI demonstrates that the fundus is barium-filled and that the duodenal bulb is air-filled. This was either an AP or a PA radiograph, which needs to be repeated. Which specific position does this radiograph represent?

_____

53. **Situation:** A patient with a clinical history of cirrhosis of the liver with acute GI bleeding comes to the radiology department. What may be the most likely reason that an esophagram was ordered for this patient?

_____

54. **Situation:** During an esophagram, the radiologist asks the patient to try to bear down as if having a bowel movement. What is this maneuver called, and why did the radiologist make such a request?

_____

55. **Situation:** During an upper GI, the radiologist reports that she sees a "lucent-halo" sign in the duodenum. What

    form of pathology did the radiologist observe? _____

56. Which one of the following technical/positioning factors does not apply to a Gastrografin® upper GI study?

    A. 125 kV   C. 40-inch (100-cm) SID

    B. Exposure made on expiration   D. Erect and recumbent positions performed

57. **Situation:** A radiograph of an upper GI is not labeled correctly, and the technologist is unsure which position was performed. A double-contrast GI study was completed with all positions performed recumbent. The radiograph demonstrates barium in the fundus and air in the body and pylorus and duodenal bulb in profile. Which position was performed?

_____

58. Which one of the following shielding devices best reduces exposure to the torso of the fluoroscopist?

    A. Lead drape   C. Lead gloves

    B. Bucky shield   D. Grid

59. **Situation:** During an esophagram, the radiologist remarks that Schatzke's ring is present. Which condition or disease process is indicated by the presence of this radiographic sign?

_____

60. **Situation:** A patient comes to radiology with a clinical history of a possible trichobezoar. What is a trichobezoar, and which radiographic procedure will best diagnose it?

_____

CHAPTER 15

Lower Gastrointestinal System

CHAPTER OBJECTIVES

After you have successfully completed the activities in this chapter, you will be able to:

_____ 1. List three divisions of the small intestine and the major parts of the large intestine.

_____ 2. Identify the function, location, and pertinent anatomy of the small and large bowel.

_____ 3. Differentiate between the terms *colon* and *large intestine*.

_____ 4. On drawings and radiographs, identify specific anatomy of the lower gastrointestinal canal from the duodenum through the anus.

_____ 5. Identify the sectional differences that differentiate the large intestine from the small intestine.

_____ 6. List specific pathologic indications and contraindications for a small bowel series and for a barium enema examination.

_____ 7. Match specific types of pathology to the correct radiographic appearances and signs.

_____ 8. Identify patient preparation for a small bowel series and for a barium enema.

_____ 9. List five safety concerns that must be followed during a barium enema procedure.

_____ 10. Identify the radiographic procedure and sequence for a small bowel series.

_____ 11. Identify the purpose, pathologic indications, and methodology for the enteroclysis and the intubation method procedures.

_____ 12. Identify the patient preparation, room preparation, and fluoroscopic procedure for a barium enema.

_____ 13. Identify the purpose, clinical indications, and methodology for an evacuative proctogram.

_____ 14. Identify the correct procedure for inserting a rectal enema tube.

_____ 15. List specific information related to the basic positions or projections of a small bowel series and barium enema examination to include size and type of image receptor, central ray location, direction and angulation of the central ray, and the anatomy best demonstrated.

_____ 16. Identify the advantages, procedure, and positioning for an air-contrast barium enema.

_____ 17. Identify patient dose ranges for skin, midline, and gonads for each small bowel and barium enema projection.

_____ 18. Given various hypothetical situations, identify the correct modification of a position and/or exposure factors to improve the radiographic image.

Positioning and Radiographic Technique

_____ 1. Using a peer, position for basic and special projections for the small bowel and barium enema series.

_____ 2. Critique and evaluate small bowel and barium enema series radiographs based on the four divisions of radiographic criteria: (1) structures shown, (2) position, (3) collimation and CR, and (4) exposure criteria.

_____ 3. Distinguish between acceptable and unacceptable small bowel and barium enema series radiographs resulting from exposure factors, motion, collimation, positioning, or other errors.

Learning Exercises

The following review exercises should be completed only after careful study of the associated pages in the textbook as indicated by each exercise. Answers to each review exercise are given at the end of the review exercises.

Part I: Radiographic Anatomy

REVIEW EXERCISE A: Radiographic Anatomy and Function of the Lower Gastrointestinal System (see textbook pp. 486-491)

1. List the three divisions of the small bowel in descending order, starting with the widest division:

    A. _____   B. _____   C. _____

2. Which division of the small bowel is the shortest? _____

3. Which division of the small bowel is the longest? _____

4. Which division of the small bowel has a feathery or coiled-spring appearance during a small bowel series?

    _____

5. A. How long is the average small bowel if removed and stretched out during autopsy? _____

    B. In a person with good muscle tone, the length of the entire small bowel is _____ .

    C. The average length of the large intestine is _____ .

6. In which two abdominal quadrants would the majority of the jejunum be found? _____

7. Which muscular band marks the junction between the duodenum and jejunum?

    _____

8. Which two aspects of the large intestine are **not** considered part of the colon? _____

9. The colon consists of _____ sections and _____ flexures.

10. List the two functions of the ileocecal valve: A. _____

    B. _____

11. What is another term for the appendix? _____

12. Match the following aspects of the small and large intestine to their characteristics:

     _____ 1. Jejunum   A. Longest aspect of the colon

     _____ 2. Duodenum   B. Widest portion of the colon

     _____ 3. Ileum   C. A blind pouch inferior to the ileocecal valve

     _____ 4. Cecum   D. Aspect of small intestine that is the smallest in diameter but longest in length

     _____ 5. Appendix   E. Distal part; also called the _iliac colon_

     _____ 6. Ascending colon   F. Shortest aspect of small intestine

     _____ 7. Descending colon   G. Lies in pelvis but possesses a wide freedom of motion

     _____ 8. Transverse colon   H. Makes up 40% of the small intestine

     _____ 9. Sigmoid colon   I. Found between the cecum and transverse colon

13. A. What is the term for the three bands of muscle that pull the large intestine into

       pouches? _____

    B. These pouches, or sacculations, seen along the large intestine wall are called _____ .

14. The part of the large intestine directly anterior to the coccyx is the _____ .

15. Identify the structures labeled on Figs. 15-1 and 15-2. Include secondary names in parentheses where indicated.

Fig. 15-1

A. _____ (_____)

B. _____

C. _____

D. _____

E. _____ (_____) _____

F. _____

G. _____ (_____) _____

H. _____

I. _____

J. _____

K. _____

L. _____

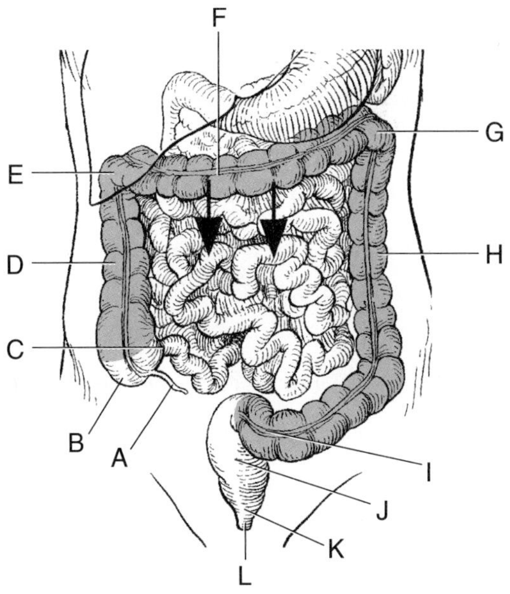

Fig. 15-1. Structures of the lower gastrointestinal tract, anterior view.

Fig. 15-2

M. _____

N. _____

O. _____

P. _____

Q. _____

R. _____

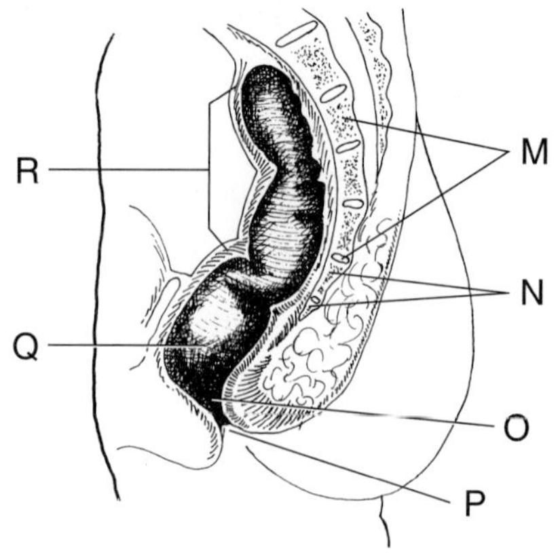

Fig. 15-2. Structures of the lower gastrointestinal tract, lateral view.

16. Which portion of the small intestine is located **primarily** to the left of the midline? _____

17. Which portion of the small intestine is located **primarily** in the RLQ? _____

18. Which portion of the small intestine has the smoothest internal lining and does **not** present a feathery appearance when barium-filled? _____

19. Which aspect of the small intestine is **most fixed** in position? _____

20. In which quadrant does the terminal ileum connect with the large intestine? _____

21. The widest portion of the large bowel is the _____.

22. Which flexure of the large bowel usually extends more superiorly? _____

23. Inflammation of the appendix is called _____.

24. Which of the following structures will fill with air during a barium enema with the patient supine? (More than one answer may be correct.)

A. Ascending colon   C. Rectum   E. Descending colon

B. Transverse colon   D. Sigmoid colon

25. Which aspect of the GI tract is primarily responsible for digestion, absorption, and reabsorption?

A. Small intestine   C. Large intestine

B. Stomach   D. Colon

26. Which aspect of the GI tract is responsible for the synthesis and absorption of vitamins B and K and amino acids?

A. Duodenum   C. Large intestine

B. Jejunum   D. Stomach

27. Four types of digestive movements occurring in the large intestine are listed below. Which one of these movement types also occurs in the small intestine?

A. Peristalsis   C. Mass peristalsis

B. Haustral churning   D. Defecation

28. Identify the gastrointestinal structures labeled on Fig. 15-3.

A. _____

B. _____

C. _____

D. _____

E. _____

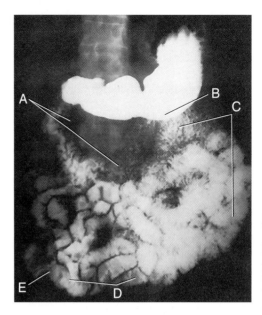

Fig. 15-3. Structure identification on a PA 30-minute small bowel radiograph.

29. Identify the gastrointestinal structures labeled on Fig. 15-4.

A. _____

B. _____

C. _____

D. _____

E. _____

F. _____

G. _____

H. _____

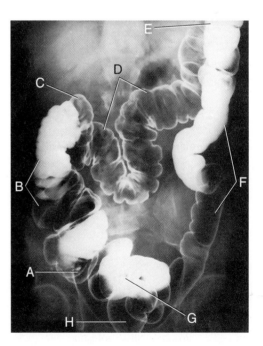

Fig. 15-4. Structure identification on an AP barium enema radiograph.

Part II: Radiographic Positioning

REVIEW EXERCISE B: Pathologic Indications and Radiographic Procedures for the Small Bowel Series and Barium Enema (see textbook pp. 492-510)

1. Which of the following conditions relates to a radiographic study of the small bowel?

A. May perform as a double-contrast media study   C. Timing of the procedure is necessary

B. An enteroclysis procedure   D. All of the above

2. Match the following definitions or statements to the correct pathologic indication for the small bowel series:

     _____ A. Common birth defect found in the ileum   1. Ileus

     _____ B. Common parasitic infection of the small intestine   2. Neoplasm

     _____ C. Obstruction of the small intestine   3. Meckel's diverticulum

     _____ D. Patient with lactose or sucrose sensitivities   4. Malabsorption syndrome

     _____ E. New growth   5. Enteritis

     _____ F. A form of sprue   6. Celiac disease

     _____ G. Inflammation of the intestine   7. Regional enteritis

     _____ H. Chronic inflammatory disease of the GI tract   8. Giardiasis

3. Match the following pathologic conditions or diseases to the correct radiographic appearance:

     _____ A. Circular staircase or herringbone sign   1. Adenocarcinoma

     _____ B. Cobblestone appearance   2. Meckel's diverticulum

     _____ C. Napkin ring sign   3. Ileus

     _____ D. Dilatation of the intestine with thickening of circular folds   4. Giardiasis

     _____ E. Large diverticulum of the ileum   5. Regional enteritis

     _____ F. "Beak sign"   6. Volvulus

4. Giardiasis is a condition acquired through:

     A. Contaminated food   C. Person-to-person contact

     B. Contaminated water   D. All of the above

5. Meckel's diverticulum is best diagnosed with which imaging modality?

     A. Small bowel series   C. Magnetic resonance imaging

     B. Enteroclysis   D. Nuclear medicine

6. Whipple's disease is a disorder of the:

     A. Distal small intestine   C. Proximal large intestine

     B. Proximal small intestine   D. Distal large intestine

7. List the two conditions that may prevent the use of barium sulfate during a small bowel series:

     A. _____   B. _____

8. What type of patients should be given extra care when using a water-soluble contrast media?

     _____

9. How much barium sulfate is generally given to an adult patient for a small-bowel-only series? _____

10. When is a small bowel series deemed completed? _____

11. How long does it usually take to complete an adult small bowel series? _____

12. When is the first radiograph generally taken during a small bowel series? _____

13. True/False: Fluoroscopy is sometimes used during a small bowel series to visualize the ileocecal valve.

14. True/False: It takes approximately 12 hours for barium sulfate, given orally, to reach the rectum.

15. The term *enteroclysis* describes what type of a small bowel study? _____

16. Which two pathologic conditions are best evaluated through an enteroclysis procedure?

    _____

17. What two types of contrast media are used for an enteroclysis?

    _____

18. The tip of the catheter is advanced to the _____ during an enteroclysis.

    A. Duodenojejunal flexure (suspensory ligament)   C. Pyloric sphincter

    B. C loop of duodenum   D. Ileocecal sphincter

19. What is the purpose of introducing methylcellulose during an enteroclysis? _____

20. A procedure to alleviate postoperative distention of a small intestine obstruction is called:

    A. Diagnostic intubation   C. Therapeutic intubation

    B. Enteroclysis   D. Small bowel series

21. What is the recommended patient preparation before a small bowel series?

    _____

22. Which position is recommended for small bowel radiographs? Why?

    _____

23. Match the following definitions or statements to the correct pathologic indication for the barium enema:

    _____ A. A twisting of a portion of the intestine on its own mesentery   1. Polyp

    _____ B. Outpouching of the mucosal wall   2. Diverticulum

    _____ C. Inflammatory condition of the large intestine   3. Intussusception

    _____ D. Severe form of colitis   4. Volvulus

    _____ E. Telescoping of one part of the intestine into another   5. Ulcerative colitis

    _____ F. Inward growth extending from the lumen of the intestinal wall   6. Colitis

24. Which type of patient usually experiences intussusception? _____

25. A condition of numerous herniations of the mucosal wall of the large intestine is called _____.

26. Which one of the following pathologic indications may produce a "tapered or corkscrew" radiographic sign during a barium enema?

   A. Diverticulosis   C. Volvulus

   B. Ulcerative colitis   D. Diverticulitis

27. Which one of the following conditions may produce the "stove pipe" radiographic sign during a barium enema?

   A. Ulcerative colitis   C. Diverticulosis

   B. Appendicitis   D. Adenocarcinoma

28. What is the most common form of carcinoma found in the large intestine?

   A. Simple-cell carcinoma   C. Annular carcinoma

   B. Basal cell carcinoma   D. Complex-cell carcinoma

29. True/False: Intestinal polyps and diverticula are very similar in structure.

30. True/False: Volvulus occurs more frequently in males than females.

31. True/False: The barium enema is a commonly recommended procedure for diagnosing possible acute appendicitis.

32. Which four conditions would prevent the use of a laxative cathartic before a barium enema procedure?

   A. _____   C. _____

   B. _____   D. _____

33. True/False: Any stool retained in the large intestine may require cancellation of a barium enema.

34. True/False: An example of an irritant cathartic is magnesium citrate.

35. True/False: Synthetic latex enema tips or gloves do not cause problems for latex-sensitive patients.

36. List the three types of enema tips commonly used (all are considered single-use and disposable):

   A. _____   B. _____   C. _____

37. What water temperature is recommended for barium enema mixtures? _____

38. To minimize spasm during a barium enema, _____ can be added to the contrast media mixture.

   A. Glucagon   C. Saline

   B. Lidocaine   D. Valium

39. What is the name of the patient position recommended for insertion of the rectal enema tip?

   _____

40. The initial insertion of the rectal enema tip should be pointed toward the:

   A. Symphysis pubis   C. Umbilicus

   B. Bladder   D. Tip of coccyx

41. Which one of the following procedures is most effective to demonstrate small polyps in the colon?

   A. Single-contrast barium enema   C. Enteroclysis

   B. Double-contrast barium enema   D. Evacuative proctogram

42. Which one of the following procedures uses the thickest mixture of barium sulfate?

     A. Single-contrast barium enema   C. Evacuative proctogram

     B. Double-contrast barium enema   D. Enteroclysis

43. Which one of the following clinical conditions is best demonstrated with evacuative proctography?

     A. Intussusception   C. Rectal prolapse

     B. Volvulus   D. Diverticulosis

44. Which aspect of the large intestine must be demonstrated during evacuative proctography?

     A. Sigmoid colon   C. Anorectal angle

     B. Haustra   D. Rectal ligament

45. Into which position is the patient placed for imaging during the evacuative proctogram?

     A. AP spine   C. Ventral decubitus

     B. Left or right lateral decubitus   D. Lateral

46. True/False: A special tapered enema tip is inserted into the stoma before a colostomy barium enema.

47. True/False: The enema bag should not be more than 36 inches (90 cm) above the table-top before the beginning of the procedure.

48. True/False: The technologist should review the patient's chart before a barium enema to determine whether a sigmoidoscopy or colonoscopy was performed recently.

49. True/False: Both computed tomography and sonography may be performed to aid in diagnosing appendicitis.

50. True/False: Because of the density and the amount of barium within the large intestine, computed radiography should not be used during a barium enema.

REVIEW EXERCISE C: Positioning of the Lower Gastrointestinal System (see textbook pp. 511-523)

1. True/False: Single-contrast barium enemas are performed commonly on patients with a clinical history of diverticula.

2. Which two special projections demonstrate the rectosigmoid region as commonly performed by 40% or more of

     clinical institutions? _____

3. The _____ projection is a recommended alternate projection for the lateral rectum with a double-contrast BE exam.

4. Where is the CR centered for the 15-minute radiograph during a small bowel series?

     A. Iliac crest   C. 2 inches (5 cm) above iliac crest

     B. Xiphoid process   D. ASIS

5. What kV is recommended for a small bowel series (with barium)? _____

6. What are the breathing instructions for a PA projection during a small bowel series?

     _____

7. Once the small bowel procedure has gone beyond 2 hours, radiographs are taken generally every _____ .

15

8. Which ionization chambers should be activated for both PA small bowel and AP and oblique barium enema projections?

     A. All three chambers   C. Left and right upper chambers

     B. Center chamber only   D. AEC should not be used for barium procedures

9. How much midline dose (also female gonadal dose) is acquired for a PA small bowel or barium enema projection of a small-to-average-size patient?

     A. 5 to 10 mrad   C. 100 to 200 mrad

     B. 30 to 50 mrad   D. 400 to 500 mrad

10. Which type of patient may require two 35- × 43-cm (14- × 17-inch) crosswise cassettes for an AP barium enema projection?

     A. Hypersthenic   C. Hyposthenic

     B. Sthenic   D. Asthenic

11. Which position(s) taken during a barium enema will best demonstrate the right colic flexure? _____

12. How much body rotation is required for oblique barium enema projections? _____

13. Which position should be performed if the patient cannot lie prone on the table to visualize the left colic flexure?

     _____

14. Which of the following barium enema positions provides the greatest amount of skin dose?

     A. Decubitus position (AP)   C. Obliques

     B. Lateral   D. AP axial

15. Which projection, taken during a double-contrast barium enema, will produce an air-filled image of the right colic flexure, ascending colon, and cecum? _____

16. Where is the CR centered for a lateral projection of the rectum? _____

17. True/False: If a retention-type enema tip is used, it should be removed after fluoroscopy is completed and prior to overhead projections are taken to better visualize the rectal region.

18. Which aspect of the large intestine is best demonstrated with an AP axial projection? _____

19. What is the advantage of performing an AP axial oblique projection rather than an AP axial?

     _____

20. A. What is another term describing the AP and PA axial projections? _____

     B. What CR angle is required for the AP axial? _____

     C. What CR angle is required for the PA axial? _____

21. Which projection during a double-contrast barium enema series best demonstrates the descending colon for possible polyps? _____

22. Which one of the following substances can be given to the patient to help stimulate evacuation following a barium enema?

     A. Milk   C. Wine or beer

     B. Coffee or hot tea   D. Garlic bread

23.   What kV range is recommended for a postevacuation projection following a barium enema? _____

24.   A.   What is the recommended kV for a single-contrast barium enema study? _____

      B.   What is the recommended kV for a double-contrast study? _____

25.   What medication can be given during a barium enema to minimize colonic spasm during a barium enema?

      _____

REVIEW EXERCISE D: Problem Solving for Technical and Positioning Errors (see textbook pp. 492-523)

1.   **Situation:** A radiograph of a double-contrast barium enema projection reveals an obscured anatomic side marker. The technologist is unsure whether it is an AP or PA recumbent projection. The transverse colon is primarily filled with barium, with the ascending and descending colon containing a lesser amount. Which position does this radiograph represent?

     _____

     _____

2.   **Situation:** A radiograph of a lateral decubitus projection taken during an air-contrast barium enema reveals that the upside aspect of the colon is overpenetrated. The following factors were used during this exposure: 120 kV, 30 mAs, 40-inch (102-cm) SID, high-speed screens, and compensating filter for the air-filled aspect of the large intestine. Which one of these factors must be modified during the repeat exposure?

     _____

     _____

3.   **Situation:** A radiograph of an AP axial barium enema projection of the rectosigmoid region reveals that there is considerable superimposition of the sigmoid colon and rectum. The following factors were used during this exposure: 120 kV, 20 mAs, 40-inch (102-cm) SID, 35° caudad CR angle, and collimation. Which one of these factors must be modified or corrected for the repeat exposure?

     _____

     _____

4.   **Situation:** A barium enema study performed on a hypersthenic patient reveals that the majority of the radiographs demonstrate that the left colic flexure was cut off. What can be done during the repeat exposures to avoid this problem?

     _____

     _____

     _____

5.   **Situation:** A technologist has inserted an air-contrast retention tip for a double-contrast BE study. He is not sure how much to inflate the retention balloon. Should he inflate it as much as the patient can tolerate, or is there a better alternative?

     _____

     _____

15

6. **Situation:** A student technologist is told to place the patient on the x-ray table in a Sims' position in preparation for the tip insertion for a barium enema. Describe how the patient should be positioned.

    _____

    _____

7. **Situation:** A patient with a clinical history of regional enteritis comes to the radiology department. What type of procedure would be most diagnostic for this condition?

    _____

    _____

8. **Situation:** A patient is referred to the radiology department for a presurgical small bowel series. What modification to the standard study needs to be made for this particular patient?

    _____

    _____

9. **Situation:** A patient comes to the radiology department for a small bowel series. However, because of a stroke, the patient is unable to swallow the contrast media. What type of study should be performed for this patient?

    _____

    _____

10. **Situation:** A young infant with a possible intussusception is brought to the emergency room. Which radiographic procedure may serve a therapeutic role in correcting this condition?

    _____

    _____

11. **Situation:** Before a barium enema, the technologist experienced difficulty in inserting the enema rectal tip (without causing significant pain for the patient). What should the technologist do to complete this task?

    _____

12. **Situation:** During the fluoroscopy aspect of a barium enema, the radiologist detects an unusual defect within the right colic flexure. She asks that the technologist provide the best images possible of this region. Which two projections will best demonstrate the right colic flexure?

    _____

13. **Situation:** A patient with a clinical history of possible enteritis comes to the radiology department. Which type of radiographic GI study would most likely be indicated for this condition? (Of course, this would have to be requested by the referring physician.)

    _____

14. **Situation:** A patient's clinical history includes possible giardiasis. What radiographic procedures would likely be indicated for this condition?

    _____

15. **Situation:** A patient came to the radiology department with a request for a small bowel series. The patient's chart indicates a possible large bowel obstruction. What radiographic exams and/or projections should be performed first before giving the patient barium to ingest for a small bowel series?

_____

_____

Part III: Laboratory Activities (see textbook pp. 511-523)

You must gain experience in positioning each part of the lower GI procedures before performing the following exams on actual patients. You can get experience in positioning and radiographic evaluation of these projections by performing exercises using radiographic phantoms and practicing on other students (although you will not be taking actual exposures).

LABORATORY EXERCISE A: Radiographic Evaluation

1. Evaluate and critique the radiographs produced during the previous experiments, additional radiographs of esophagrams and lower GI procedures provided by your instructor, or both. Evaluate each position for the following points (check off when completed):

   _____ Evaluate the completeness of the study. (Are all of the pertinent anatomic structures included on the radiograph?)

   _____ Evaluate for positioning or centering errors (e.g., rotation, off centering)

   _____ Evaluate for correct exposure factors and possible motion. (Are the density and contrast of the images acceptable?)

   _____ Determine whether markers and an acceptable degree of collimation and/or area shielding are visible on the images.

LABORATORY EXERCISE B: Physical Positioning

On another person, simulate performing all basic and special projections of the lower GI as follows. Include the six steps listed below and described in the textbook. (Check off each when completed satisfactorily.)

Step 1. Appropriate size and type of image receptor (IR) with correct markers
Step 2. Correct CR placement and centering of part to CR and/or IR
Step 3. Accurate collimation
Step 4. Area shielding of patient where advisable
Step 5. Use of proper immobilizing devices when needed
Step 6. Approximate correct exposure factors, breathing instructions where applicable, and "making" exposure

	STEP 1	STEP 2	STEP 3	STEP 4	STEP 5	STEP 6
• PA 15- or 30-minute small bowel	_____	_____	_____	_____	_____	_____
• PA 1- or 2-hour small bowel	_____	_____	_____	_____	_____	_____
• PA or AP barium enema	_____	_____	_____	_____	_____	_____
• RAO and LAO barium enema	_____	_____	_____	_____	_____	_____
• LPO and RPO barium enema	_____	_____	_____	_____	_____	_____
• Right and left lateral decubitus	_____	_____	_____	_____	_____	_____
• AP and LPO axial	_____	_____	_____	_____	_____	_____
• PA and RAO axial	_____	_____	_____	_____	_____	_____
• Lateral rectum	_____	_____	_____	_____	_____	_____
• Ventral decubitus lateral rectum	_____	_____	_____	_____	_____	_____

15

Answers to Review Exercises

Review Exercise A: Radiographic Anatomy and Function of the Lower Gastrointestinal System

1. A. Duodenum
   B. Jejunum
   C. Ileum
2. Duodenum
3. Ileum
4. Jejunum
5. A. 23 feet, or 7 m
   B. 15 to 18 feet, or 4.5 to 5.5 m
   C. 5 feet, or 1.5 m
6. LUQ and LLQ
7. Suspensory ligament of the duodenum or ligament of Treitz (this site is a reference point for certain small bowel exams because it remains in a relatively fixed position)
8. Cecum and rectum
9. 4 sections; 2 flexures
10. A. Prevents contents of the ileum from passing too quickly into cecum
    B. Prevents reflux back into the ileum
11. Vermiform appendix
12. 1. H, 2. F, 3. D, 4. B, 5. C, 6. I, 7. E, 8. A, 9. G
13. A. Taeniae coli
    B. Haustra
14. Rectal ampulla
15. A. Vermiform appendix (appendix)
    B. Cecum
    C. Ileocecal valve
    D. Ascending colon
    E. Right colic (hepatic) flexure
    F. Transverse colon
    G. Left colic (splenic) flexure
    H. Descending colon
    I. Sigmoid colon
    J. Rectum
    K. Anal canal
    L. Anus
    M. Sacrum
    N. Coccyx
    O. Anal canal
    P. Anus
    Q. Rectal ampulla
    R. Rectum
16. Jejunum
17. Ileum
18. Ileum
19. Duodenojejunal junction
20. Right lower quadrant (RLQ)
21. Cecum
22. Left colic (splenic)
23. Appendicitis
24. B. Transverse colon
    D. Sigmoid colon

25. A. Small intestine
26. C. Large intestine
27. A. Peristalsis
28. A. Duodenum
    B. Area of suspensory ligament/duodenojejunal junction
    C. Jejunum
    D. Ileum
    E. Area of ileocecal valve
29. A. Cecum
    B. Ascending colon
    C. Right colic (hepatic) flexure
    D. Transverse colon
    E. Left colic (splenic) flexure
    F. Descending colon
    G. Sigmoid colon
    H. Rectum

Review Exercise B: Pathologic Indications and Radiographic Procedures for the Small Bowel Series and Barium Enema

1. D. All of the above
2. A. 3
   B. 8
   C. 1
   D. 4
   E. 2
   F. 6
   G. 5
   H. 7
3. A. 3
   B. 5
   C. 1
   D. 4
   E. 2
   F. 6
4. D. All of the above
5. D. Nuclear medicine
6. B. Proximal small intestine
7. A. Possible perforated hollow viscus
   B. Large bowel obstruction
8. Young and dehydrated
9. 2 cups, or 16 ounces
10. When the contrast medium passes through the ileocecal valve
11. 2 hours
12. 15 to 30 minutes after ingesting the contrast medium
13. True
14. False (24 hours)
15. Double-contrast method
16. Regional enteritis (Crohn's disease) and malabsorption syndromes
17. High-density barium sulfate and air or methylcellulose
18. A. Duodenojejunal flexure (suspensory ligament)

19. It dilates the intestinal lumen to produce a more diagnostic study
20. C. Therapeutic intubation
21. NPO for at least 8 hours before procedure; no smoking or gum chewing
22. Prone. To separate the loops of bowel
23. A. 4
    B. 2
    C. 6
    D. 5
    E. 3
    F. 1
24. Infant
25. Diverticulosis
26. C. Volvulus
27. A. Ulcerative colitis
28. C. Annular carcinoma
29. False
30. True
31. False
32. A. Gross bleeding
    B. Severe diarrhea
    C. Obstruction
    D. Inflammatory lesions
33. True
34. False (castor oil is an irritant cathartic)
35. True
36. A. Plastic disposable
    B. Rectal retention
    C. Air-contrast retention
37. Room temperature (85 to 90 degrees)
38. B. Lidocaine
39. Sims' position
40. C. Umbilicus
41. B. Double-contrast barium enema
42. C. Evacuative proctogram
43. C. Rectal prolapse
44. C. Anorectal angle
45. D. Lateral
46. True
47. False (not more than 24 inches [60 cm] above tabletop when beginning the procedure)
48. True
49. True
50. False

Review Exercise C: Positioning of the Lower Gastrointestinal System

1. False
2. AP or PA axial (butterfly)
3. Ventral decubitus
4. C. 2 inches (5 cm) above iliac crest
5. 100 to 125 kV

15

6. Make exposure on expiration.
7. Hour
8. A. All three chambers
9. B. 30 to 50 mrad
10. A. Hypersthenic
11. RAO or LPO
12. 35° to 45°
13. RPO
14. B. Lateral
15. Left lateral decubitus
16. Level of ASIS at the midcoronal plane
17. False (generally should not be removed until after overhead projections are completed unless directed to do so by the radiologist)
18. Rectosigmoid region
19. Creates less superimposition of the rectosigmoid segments
20. A. Butterfly projections
    B. AP: CR angled 30° to 40° cephalad
    C. PA: CR 30° to 40° caudad
21. Right lateral decubitus (left side up)
22. B. Coffee or hot tea
23. 80 to 90 kV
24. A. 100 to 125 kV
    B. 80 to 90 kV
25. Glucagon

Review Exercise D: Problem Solving for Technical and Positioning Errors

1. PA prone. Since the transverse colon is an intraperitoneal aspect of the large intestine located more anteriorly, it will fill with barium in the PA prone position.
2. Even with the use of a compensating filter, a reduction in kV is required. Since less barium sulfate is used during an air-contrast procedure, the kV range should be 80 to 90.
3. The CR was angled in the wrong direction. The AP axial projection requires a 30° to 40° cephalad angle.
4. Use two 14- × 17-inch (35- × 43-cm) crosswise cassettes for the AP/PA and oblique projections, one centered higher and one lower. Since hypersthenic patients have a wider distribution of the large intestine, two crosswise-placed cassettes will ensure that all of the pertinent anatomy is demonstrated.
5. Retention catheters should be fully inflated only by the radiologist under fluoroscopic control.
6. Lay on left side and flex head and upper body forward, drawing the right leg up above the partially flexed left leg.
7. Enteroclysis, a double-contrast small bowel procedure. A basic small bowel series may also demonstrate this condition, but the enteroclysis with double contrast is more effective in demonstrating mucosal changes.
8. Since the patient is having surgery soon after the small bowel series, a water-soluble, iodinated contrast media should be used. Barium sulfate should not be given to presurgical patients.
9. A diagnostic intubation small bowel series would be preferred. A nasogastric tube would be passed into the small intestine, allowing the contrast media to be instilled. This procedure is effective for patients who can't swallow.
10. A barium enema or air enema often leads to re-expansion of the telescoped aspect of the large intestine (see textbook, p. 499)
11. Inform the radiologist and have him or her insert it under fluoroscopic guidance
12. RAO or LPO projections
13. A small bowel series (Enteritis is an inflammation or infection of the small intestine.)
14. An upper GI, small bowel combination series (Gastroenteritis is an inflammation or infection of both the stomach and small intestine.)
15. An acute abdominal series and a barium enema to rule out a possible large bowel obstruction (Barium by mouth is contraindicated with a possible large bowel obstruction.)

SELF-TEST

My Score = _____ %

Directions: This self-test should be taken only after completing all of the readings, review exercises, and laboratory activities for a particular section. The purpose of this test is not only to provide a good learning exercise but also to serve as a good indicator of what your final evaluation exam will be. It is strongly suggested that if you do not get at least a 90% to 95% grade on each self-test, you review those areas in which you missed questions before going to your instructor for the final evaluation exam for this chapter. (There are 78 questions or blanks—each is worth 1.3 points.)

1. During life, how long is the entire small intestine?

    A. 15 to 18 feet (4.5 to 5.5 m)   C. 5 to 10 feet (1.5 to 3 m)

    B. 20 to 25 feet (6 to 7.5 m)   D. 30 to 40 feet (9 to 12 m)

2. Which aspect of the small intestine is considered the longest?

    A. Duodenum   C. Ileum

    B. Jejunum   D. Cecum

3. What is the name for the band of muscular tissue found at the junction of the duodenum and jejunum?

    A. Valvulae conniventes   C. Duodenal flexure

    B. Haustra   D. Suspensory ligament of the duodenum

4. Which aspect of the small intestine possesses the smallest diameter?

    A. Ileum   C. Cecum

    B. Duodenum   D. Jejunum

5. The part of the intestine with a "feathery" and "coiled spring" appearance when filled with barium is the:

    A. Ileum   C. Jejunum

    B. Duodenum   D. Cecum

6. List the two aspects of the large intestine not considered part of the colon.

    A. _____   B. _____

7. What is the correct term for the appendix? _____

8. True/False: The rectum possesses two anteroposterior curves that have a direct impact on rectal enema tip insertions.

9. True/False: The small sacculations found within the jejunum are called *haustra*.

10. Which colic flexure (**right** or **left**) is located 1 to 2 inches (2.5 to 5 cm) higher or more superior in the abdomen?

    _____

15

11. Identify the labeled structures on the following radiographs (Figs. 15-5 and 15-6). Include secondary names where indicated by parentheses.

Fig.15-5:

A. _____

B. _____

C. _____

D. _____

E. _____

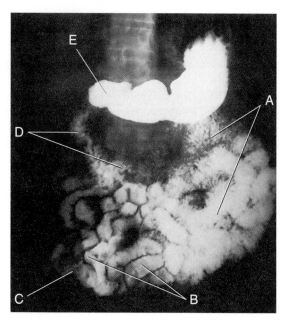

Fig. 15-5. Structure identification on a gastrointestinal radiograph.

Fig.15-6:

F. _____ (_____) _____

G. _____

H. _____

I. _____

J. _____

K. _____

L. _____ (_____) _____

M. _____

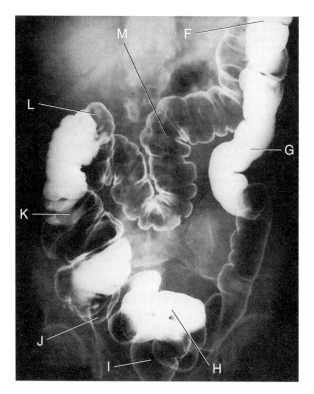

Fig. 15-6. Structure identification on a barium enema radiograph.

12. Which one of the following structures is considered to be most anterior?

A. Cecum C. Transverse colon

B. Rectum D. Ascending colon

13.   Where does the reabsorption of inorganic salts occur in the gastrointestinal tract?

A.   Duodenum   C.   Stomach

B.   Large intestine   D.   Jejunum

14.   Which one of the following digestive movements occurs in the small intestine?

A.   Haustral churning   C.   Mass peristalsis

B.   Rhythmic segmentation   D.   Mastication

15.   Match each of the following pathologic indications to its correct definition:

_____   1.   Meckel's diverticulum   A.   Telescoping of the bowel into another aspect of it

_____   2.   Diverticulosis   B.   A new growth extending from mucosal wall

_____   3.   Enteritis   C.   A twisting of the intestine on its own mesentery

_____   4.   Whipple's disease   D.   Condition of small herniations present along the intestinal wall

_____   5.   Polyp   E.   Chronic inflammatory condition of small intestine

_____   6.   Malabsorption syndrome   F.   Outpouching located in distal ileum

_____   7.   Diverticulitis   G.   Unable to process certain nutrients

_____   8.   Volvulus   H.   May be caused by cutting off blood supply to it or infection

_____   9.   Intussusception   I.   Inflammation of the small intestine

_____ 10.   Regional enteritis   J.   Inflammation of small herniations in the intestinal wall

_____ 11.   Ulcerative colitis   K.   Caused by a flagellate protozoan

_____ 12.   Giardiasis   L.   Disorder of proximal small intestine

_____ 13.   Appendicitis   M.   Chronic inflammatory condition of the large intestine

16.   Match the following radiographic appearances to the correct pathologic indication:

_____   1.   A tapered or corkscrew appearance seen during a barium enema   A.   Ulcerative colitis

_____   2.   Apple-core lesion   B.   Diverticulosis

_____   3.   String sign   C.   Intussusception

_____   4.   Dilatation of the intestine with thickening of the circular folds   D.   Volvulus

_____   5.   Stove-pipe appearance of colon   E.   Regional enteritis

_____   6.   Mushroom-shaped dilatation with a small amount of barium
              extending beyond it   F.   Polyp

                                                                                     G.   Neoplasm

_____   7.   Jagged or sawtooth appearance of the intestinal mucosa

                                                                                     H.   Giardiasis

_____   8.   Inward growth from intestinal wall

17. Which of the following imaging modalities/procedures is often performed to diagnose and may treat an intussusception?

    A. Barium enema   C. Nuclear medicine scan

    B. Enteroclysis   D. CT

18. True/False: The barium enema is recommended to diagnose acute appendicitis.

19. What breathing instructions should be given to the patient during insertion of the enema tip?

    _____

20. Why is the PA rather than AP recumbent position recommended for a small bowel series?

    _____

21. What is the minimum amount of time a patient needs to remain NPO before a small bowel series? _____

22. What is another term for a laxative? _____

23. Which type of rectal enema tip is ideal for the patient with a relaxed anal sphincter?

    _____

24. What is the name of the drug that can be given to help control intestinal spasm during a barium enema?

    _____

25. What drug can be added to the barium sulfate mixture to minimize intestinal spasm during a barium enema?

    _____

26. Which one of the following pathologic indications is best diagnosed during an evacuative proctogram?

    A. Regional enteritis   C. Volvulus

    B. Diverticulosis   D. Prolapse of rectum

27. Which region of the large intestine must be visualized during an evacuative proctogram study?

    A. Cecum   C. Ileocecal valve

    B. Anorectal angle   D. Left colic flexure

28. True/False: A small balloon retention catheter may be placed within the stoma of the colostomy to deliver contrast media during a barium enema.

29. Which oblique position, the LAO or RAO, best demonstrates the ascending colon and cecum? _____

30. What is the average length of time in a routine small bowel series for the barium pass through the ileocecal sphincter?

    _____

31. Which one of the following commercial contrast media would be used during an evaluative proctogram?

    A. Hypaque   C. Gastroview

    B. Gastrografin   D. Anatrast

32.   Which ionization chambers should be activated for a lateral barium enema projection of the rectum?

    A. All three chambers   C. Center chamber only

    B. Right and left upper chambers   D. Right upper chamber only

33.   How much rotation of the body is required for the LAO position during a barium enema? _____

34.   The CR and image receptor should be centered about _____ higher for the 15- or

    30-minute small bowel image than for the later images.

35.   The term *evacuative proctography* is sometimes used for a lower GI tract procedure. This procedure is also

    commonly called _____ .

36.   **Situation:** A patient is unable to lie prone on the radiographic table during a barium enema. Which specific

    position will best demonstrate the right colic flexure? _____

37.   **Situation:** A patient is scheduled for an air-contrast barium enema. During the fluoroscopy phase of the study, the
    radiologist detects a possible polyp in the lower descending colon. Which specific position will best demonstrate
    this region of the colon?

    _____

    _____

38.   **Situation:** A patient with a clinical history of a rectocele comes to the radiology department. Which radiographic

    procedure will best diagnose this condition? _____

39.   True/False: A PA axial oblique (RAO) barium enema projection is an optional projection to demonstrate the right
    colic flexure.

40.   True/False: On a hypersthenic-type patient, a 35- × 43-cm (14- × 17-inch) IR placed lengthwise and centered
    correctly will generally include the entire barium-filled large intestine on one IR.

41.   True/False: The female gonadal dose for a lateral barium enema projection is approximately 15 to 20 times greater
    than for a lateral decubitus (AP) projection.

42.   The skin dose range for a lateral rectum position on an average-size patient is:

    A. 50 to 100 mrad   C. 500 to 1000 mrad

    B. 200 to 400 mrad   D. 2000 to 3000 mrad

43.   A. The RAO position best demonstrates the _____ (**right** or **left**) colic flexure with the

       CR and image receptor centered to the level of _____ .

    B. The LAO position best demonstrates the _____ (**right** or **left**) colic flexure with the

       CR and image receptor centered to the level of _____ .

15

44.   True/False: Latex-based gloves are safe to be worn by all technologists.

45.   **Situation:** During a barium enema, a possible polyp is seen in the left colic flexure. Which of the following positions will best demonstrate it?

      A.   RPO   C.   RAO

      B.   AP axial   D.   PA

46.   **Situation:** A patient has a clinical history of regional enteritis. Which of the following procedures is most often performed for this condition?

      A.   Intubation small bowel series   C.   Enteroclysis

      B.   Single-contrast barium enema   D.   Double-contrast barium enema

47.   **Situation:** A patient comes to the radiology department with a clinical history of Meckel's diverticulum. Which

      imaging modality is most often performed for this condition? _____

48.   **Situation:** A patient comes to the radiology department with a clinical history of giardiasis. She is scheduled for a barium enema procedure. Which of the following precautions must be followed during the procedure?

      A.   Wear gloves   C.   Wear eye protection

      B.   Wear surgical mask   D.   All of the above

49.   _____ is a group of intestinal malabsorption diseases involving the inability to absorb certain proteins and dietary fat.

50.   True/False: The transit time of barium through the small intestine of the pediatric patient is less than that required for an adult.

CHAPTER 16

Gallbladder and Biliary Ducts

After you have successfully completed the activities in this chapter, you will be able to:

_____ 1. Identify specific anatomy and functions of the liver, gallbladder, and biliary ductal system.

_____ 2. Describe the production, storage, and purpose of bile.

_____ 3. On drawings and radiographs, identify specific anatomy of the biliary system.

_____ 4. Describe the effect of body habitus on the location of the gallbladder.

_____ 5. Define specific terms related to conditions and procedures of the biliary system.

_____ 6. Define specific pathologies of the biliary system.

_____ 7. Match specific biliary pathologies to the correct radiographic appearances and signs.

_____ 8. Identify special and alternative radiographic procedures of the biliary system.

_____ 9. List the advantages of ultrasound of the gallbladder as compared with the oral cholecystogram.

_____ 10. List information related to the percutaneous transhepatic, T-tube, and endoscopic retrograde cholangiopancreatogram procedures, including purpose of study, contraindications, imaging, and postprocedure care.

_____ 11. List information related to the basic and special projections for an oral cholecystogram, including size and type of image receptor (IR), central ray location, direction and angulation of the central ray, and anatomy best visualized.

_____ 12. Identify the patient dose ranges for skin, midline, and gonads for various oral cholecystogram projections.

_____ 13. Given various hypothetical situations, identify the correct modification of a position and/or exposure factors to improve the radiographic image.

Positioning and Radiographic Critique

_____ 1. Using a peer, position for basic and special projections for an oral cholecystogram procedure.

_____ 2. Critique and evaluate oral cholecystogram and cholangiogram radiographs based on the four divisions of radiographic criteria: (1) structures shown, (2) position, (3) collimation and CR, and (4) exposure criteria.

_____ 3. Distinguish between acceptable and unacceptable biliary study radiographs resulting from exposure factors, motion, collimation, positioning, or other errors.

Learning Exercises

The following review exercises should be completed only after careful study of the associated pages in the textbook as indicated by each exercise. Answers to each review exercise are given at the end of the review exercises.

Part I: Radiographic Anatomy

REVIEW EXERCISE A: Radiographic Anatomy of the Gallbladder and Biliary System (see textbook pp. 526-528)

1. What is the average weight of the adult human liver? _____

2. Which abdominal quadrant contains the gallbladder? _____

3. What is the name of the soft-tissue structure that separates the right from the left lobe of the liver?

    _____

4. Which lobe of the liver is larger, the right or left? _____

5. List the other two lobes of the liver (in addition to right and left lobes):

    A. _____   B. _____

6. True/False: The liver performs over 100 functions.

7. True/False: The average healthy adult liver produces 1 gallon, or 3000 to 4000 ml, of bile per day.

8. List the three primary functions of the gallbladder:

    A. _____

    B. _____

    C. _____

9. True/False: Concentrated levels of cholesterol in bile may lead to gallstones.

10. What is a common site for impaction, or lodging, of gallstones? _____

11. True/False: In about 40% of individuals, the end of the common bile duct and the end of the pancreatic duct are totally separated into two ducts rather than combining into one single passageway into the duodenum.

12. True/False: An older term for the main pancreatic duct is *the duct of Vater*.

13. The gallbladder is located more _____ (**posteriorly** or **anteriorly**) within the abdomen.

14. Match the following structures to their primary location within the abdomen.

    _____ 1. Liver   A. Near midsagittal plane

    _____ 2. Gallbladder on asthenic patient   B. To left of midsagittal plane

    _____ 3. Gallbladder on hypersthenic patient   C. To right of midsagittal plane

    _____ 4. Gallbladder on hyposthenic patient

16

15. Identify the major components of the gallbladder and biliary system labeled on Fig. 16-1:

A. _____

B. _____

C. _____

D. _____

E. _____

F. _____

G. _____

H. _____

I. _____

J. _____

K. _____

L. _____

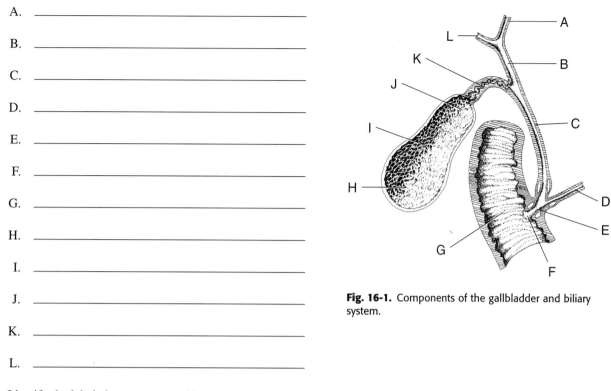

Fig. 16-1. Components of the gallbladder and biliary system.

16. Identify the labeled structures on this sagittal view of the abdomen (Fig. 16-2):

A. _____

B. _____

C. _____

D. _____

E. _____

F. _____

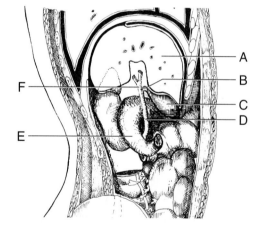

Fig. 16-2. Sagittal, cut-away view of components of the gallbladder and biliary system.

17. In what position should the patient be placed if the primary purpose is to drain the gallbladder into the duct system?

_____

18. Which projection (AP or PA) would place the gallbladder closest to the IR for the best visualization? _____

19. Which radiographic oblique position will project the gallbladder away from the spine? _____

Part II: Radiographic Positioning

REVIEW EXERCISE B: Radiographic Procedures and Positioning of the Gallbladder and Biliary Ducts (see textbook pp. 529-541)

1. The prefix *chole* refers to _____ .

2. The prefix *cysto* refers to _____ .

3. Radiographic examination of the gallbladder is called _____ .

4. Radiographic examination of the biliary ducts is called _____ .

5. Radiographic examination of both the gallbladder and biliary ducts is called _____ .

6. The acronym *OCG* refers to _____ .

7. Oral types of contrast media designed to visualize the gallbladder are called _____ .

8. List the three biliary functions measured during an OCG:

    A. _____

    B. _____

    C. _____

9. In addition to hypersensitivity to iodinated compounds, what are the three other contraindications to an OCG?

    A. _____   C. _____

    B. _____

10. Match each of the following pathologic indications with its correct definition:

    _____ 1. Cholelithiasis   A. Defects present at birth

    _____ 2. Cholecystitis   B. Emulsion of biliary stones

    _____ 3. Biliary stenosis   C. Condition of having gallstones

    _____ 4. Congenital anomalies   D. Inflammation of the gallbladder

    _____ 5. Neoplasm   E. Benign or malignant tumors

    _____ 6. Milk calcium bile   F. Narrowing of the biliary ducts

11. True/False: The majority of gallstones contain enough calcium to be visualized on a plain abdomen radiograph.

12. True/False: Chronic cholecystitis is usually associated with gallstones.

13. True/False: Acute cholecystitis may produce a thickened gallbladder wall.

14. True/False: A nonvisualized gallbladder during an OCG is always the result of a pathologic condition.

15. True/False: The patient must take laxatives 8 hours before an OCG to ensure that the colon is free of feces, which may obscure the gallbladder.

16

16. True/False: Patients on a fat-free diet should eat some fat 1 or 2 days before an OCG exam.

17. True/False: Most disorders of the gallbladder and biliary duct are caused by gallstones.

18. How many hours before an OCG should the cholecystopaques be taken? _____

19. What is the optimal kV range for an OCG? _____

20. What five questions should a patient be asked before the cholecystogram scout is taken?

    A. _____

    B. _____

    C. _____

    E. (Female patient) _____

21. True/False: The RAO is the most important position for imaging the gallbladder.

22. What type of needle is used during a PTC? _____

23. List four advantages of a gallbladder ultrasound instead of the conventional OCG:

    A. _____

    B. _____

    C. _____

    D. _____

24. Postoperative (T-tube) cholangiograms are usually performed to detect:

    A. Pancreatitis   C. Liver cyst

    B. Biliary stones   D. Infected gallbladder

25. True/False: A PTC is usually performed by a surgeon.

26. Postoperative (T-tube) cholangiograms are generally performed _____ (**during surgery** or **in the radiology department**).

27. Which one of the following procedures may be performed during a postoperative (T-tube) cholangiogram?

    A. Remove the gallbladder   C. Remove a biliary stone

    B. Remove a liver cyst   D. Catheterize the hepatic portal vein

28. Which one of the following clinical conditions is best suited for a percutaneous cholangiogram (PTC)?

    A. Obstructive jaundice   C. Liver hemorrhage

    B. Ascites   D. Cholelithiasis

29. Why is a chest radiograph commonly ordered following a PTC? _____

30. Which one of the following is not an expected risk associated with a PTC?

    A. Liver hemorrhage   C. Escape of bile

    B. Pneumothorax   D. Cholecystitis

16

31.   A.   A radiographic procedure of examining the biliary and main pancreatic ducts is called a(n)

_____ (write out full term).

   B.   What initials are commonly used as an abbreviation for this procedure? _____

   C.   What type of special endoscope is commonly used for this procedure? _____

   D.   Which member of the health care team usually performs this procedure? _____

   E.   Why should a patient remain NPO at least 1 hour following this procedure? _____

32.   Match each of the following biliary procedures with the means of introducing the contrast media during that procedure:

_____ 1. ERCP

_____ 2. PTC

_____ 3. T-tube cholangiogram

_____ 4. Immediate cholangiogram

_____ 5. OCG

_____ 6. Cholecystosonography

A.   Direct injection through a catheter placed during an endoscopic process

B.   No contrast media required

C.   Oral ingestion

D.   Direct injection by a needle

E.   Direct injection through indwelling drainage tube puncture

F.   Direct injection through catheter during surgery

33.   True/False: Conditions such as sickle cell anemia may produce gallstones in pediatric patients.

34.   True/False: HIDA nuclear medicine scans are primarily performed to diagnose cirrhosis of the liver.

35.   Which imaging modality/procedure is recommended for a gallbladder study on a pediatric patient?

   A. OCG   C. MRI

   B. Sonography   D. CT

36.   True/False: Gallbladder projections result in approximately equal levels of gonadal dose for males and females.

37.   True/False: The right upper AEC ionization chamber is recommended for gallbladder projections.

38.   The gallbladder is usually found on the sthenic patient at the vertebral level of:

   A. T12   B. L4   C. T10   D. L2

39.   Centering for a PA scout projection on a hypersthenic patient is usually _____ as compared with a sthenic patient.

   A.   Lower and more midline   C.   Higher and midline

   B.   About the same location   D.   Higher and more lateral

40.   Which oblique position will project the gallbladder away from the spine? _____

41.   How much rotation of the body is required for this projection taken on (A) an asthenic patient? _____

   (B) a hypersthenic patient? _____

42.   Which two possible positions during an OCG will stratify any possible gallstones?

   A. _____   B. _____

43.   Which specific decubitus position should be performed to demonstrate possible stratification (layering out) of

gallstones? _____

44.   What is the gonadal dose given to a female patient with a decubitus projection during an OCG?

A.   Not measurable   C.   50 to 100 mrad

B.   5 to 10 mrad   D.   200 to 400 mrad

45.   How much lower should centering be for an erect gallbladder projection as compared with a recumbent projection?

_____

REVIEW EXERCISE C: Problem Solving for Technical and Positioning Errors (see textbook pp. 529-541)

1.   **Situation:** An asthenic-type patient comes to the radiology department for an oral cholecystogram. The PA scout
projection fails to reveal the location of the gallbladder. The following factors were used during the initial exposure:
10- × 12-inch (24- × 30-cm) lengthwise IR, 70 kV, 30 mAs, 40-inch (102-cm) SID, Bucky, CR centered to the level
of L2. Which of these factors can be modified to increase the chances of locating the gallbladder?

_____

_____

2.   **Situation:** A radiograph of a PA scout projection for an OCG reveals that the gallbladder is only faintly visible.
The patient assures the technologist that she took all the required tablets. The following factors were used during
the exposure: 85 kV, AEC with center cell, Bucky, CR centered to the level of L2. Which of these factors can be
modified to improve the visibility of the gallbladder?

_____

_____

3.   **Situation:** A radiograph of an LAO projection reveals that the gallbladder is superimposed over the spine. What
type of positioning modification is needed to prevent this superimposition during the repeat exposure?

_____

_____

4.   **Situation:** During an operative cholangiogram, the resultant radiograph reveals that the biliary ducts are
superimposed over the spine. As requested by the surgeon, the initial projection was taken AP in the supine
position. What can be done to shift the biliary ducts away from the spine during the repeat exposure?

_____

_____

5.   **Situation:** A patient with right upper quadrant pain enters the emergency room. The physician is concerned about
gallstones, but the patient states that he is hypersensitive to iodine. Which procedure of the biliary system would be
ideal for this patient?

_____

_____

16

6. **Situation:** A patient with signs of obstructive jaundice enters the emergency room. The patient's skin has a yellow tinge to it. Which radiographic study of the biliary system would be recommended for this patient?

_____

_____

7. **Situation:** A patient comes to radiology with a clinical history of cholelithiasis. A previous OCG did not visualize the gallbladder. The referring physician is more concerned about the function of the gallbladder. What other imaging modality will demonstrate both anatomy and function of the gallbladder?

_____

_____

8. **Situation:** A patient who may have a stone in the main pancreatic duct enters the emergency room. Other than sonography, which procedure would be ideal to demonstrate this duct and determine whether a stone is present?

_____

9. **Situation:** A patient with a history of acute cholecystitis comes to the radiology department for an OCG. The scout image does not demonstrate an opacified gallbladder. What other procedure(s) can be ordered to visualize the gallbladder and biliary ducts?

_____

10. **Situation:** A patient who may have a neoplasm of the gallbladder comes to the radiology department. Which imaging modalities or procedures would best diagnose this condition?

_____

16

Part III: Laboratory Exercises (see textbook pp. 529-541)

Although it is impossible to duplicate many aspects of biliary studies on a phantom in the laboratory, evaluation of actual radiographs and physical positioning is possible. You can get experience in positioning and radiographic evaluation of these projections by performing exercises using radiographic phantoms and practicing on other students (although you will not be taking actual exposures). Technologists must learn the positioning routine, room setup, and fluoroscopy procedure for their particular facility.

LABORATORY EXERCISE A: Radiographic Evaluation

Using actual radiographs of OCG and cholangiogram procedures provided by your instructor, evaluate and critique each position for the following points (check off when completed):

_____   Evaluate the completeness of the study. (Are all of the pertinent anatomic structures included on the radiograph?)

_____   Evaluate for positioning or centering errors (e.g., rotation, off centering).

_____   Evaluate for correct exposure factors and possible motion. (Is the contrast medium properly penetrated?)

_____   Determine whether patient obliquity is correct for specific positions.

_____   Determine whether markers and an acceptable degree of collimation and/or area shielding are visible on
the images.

LABORATORY EXERCISE B: Physical Positioning

On another person, simulate performing all basic and special projections of an OCG as follows. Include the six steps listed
below and described in the textbook. (Check off each when completed satisfactorily.)

Step 1. Appropriate size and type of image receptor with correct markers
Step 2. Correct CR placement and centering of part to CR and/or image receptor
Step 3. Accurate collimation
Step 4. Area shielding of patient where advisable
Step 5. Use of proper immobilizing devices when needed
Step 6. Approximate correct exposure factors, breathing instructions where applicable, and "making" exposure

PROJECTIONS	STEP 1	STEP 2	STEP 3	STEP 4	STEP 5	STEP 6
• PA scout	_____	_____	_____	_____	_____	_____
• LAO	_____	_____	_____	_____	_____	_____
• Right lateral decubitus	_____	_____	_____	_____	_____	_____
• PA erect	_____	_____	_____	_____	_____	_____
Optional:						
• RPO for biliary ducts	_____	_____	_____	_____	_____	_____

16

Answers to Review Exercises

Review Exercise A: Radiographic Anatomy of the Gallbladder and Biliary System
1. 3 to 4 pounds (1.5 kg), or ¹⁄₆₀ of total body weight
2. Right upper quadrant (RUQ)
3. Falciform ligament
4. Right
5. A. Quadrate
   B. Caudate
6. True
7. False (1 quart, or 800 to 1000 ml)
8. A. Store bile
   B. Concentrate bile
   C. Contract to release bile into duodenum
9. True
10. Duodenal papilla
11. True
12. False (duct of Wirsung)
13. Anteriorly
14. 1. C
    2. A
    3. C
    4. C
15. A. Left hepatic duct
    B. Common hepatic duct
    C. Common bile duct
    D. Pancreatic duct
    E. Hepatopancreatic ampulla (ampulla of Vater)
    F. Duodenal papilla
    G. Duodenum
    H. Fundus of gallbladder
    I. Body of gallbladder
    J. Neck of gallbladder
    K. Cystic duct
    L. Right hepatic duct
16. A. Liver
    B. Cystic duct
    C. Gallbladder
    D. Common bile duct
    E. Duodenum
    F. Common hepatic duct
17. Supine
18. PA
19. LAO

Review Exercise B: Radiographic Procedures and Positioning of the Gallbladder and Biliary Ducts
1. Bile
2. Bladder or sac
3. Cholecystography
4. Cholangiography
5. Cholecystocholangiography
6. Oral cholecystogram
7. Cholecystopaques
8. A. Functional ability of the liver to remove contrast media
   B. Patency and condition of the biliary ducts
   C. Concentrating and contracting ability of the gallbladder
9. A. Advanced hepatorenal disease
   B. Active gastrointestinal disease
   C. Pregnancy
10. 1. C
    2. D
    3. F
    4. A
    5. E
    6. B
11. False (only about 15% are visualized)
12. True
13. True
14. False (may be other reasons)
15. False (NPO 8 hrs)
16. True
17. True
18. 10 to 12 hours before the procedure
19. 70 to 80 kV
20. A. How many pills were taken and at what time?
    B. Any reaction from the pills?
    C. Did you have breakfast?
    D. Do you still have your gallbladder?
    E. Is there a possibility of pregnancy?
21. False
22. Chiba (or "skinny") needle
23. A. No ionizing radiation
    B. Better detection of small calculi
    C. No contrast media required
    D. Less time-consuming procedure
24. B. Biliary stones
25. False
26. In the radiology department
27. C. Remove a biliary stone
28. A. Obstructive jaundice
29. Rule out a possible pneumothorax
30. D. Cholecystitis
31. A. Endoscopic retrograde cholangiopancreatogram
    B. ERCP
    C. Duodenoscope or video endoscope
    D. Gastroenterologist
    E. Prevent aspiration of food or liquid into the lungs
32. 1. A
    2. D
    3. E
    4. F
    5. C
    6. B
33. True
34. False (HIDA scans are a study of the gallbladder and biliary ducts.)
35. B. Sonography
36. False (female ≈6 mrad; males 0.1 mrad)
37. False (The center chamber should be used.)
38. D. L2
39. D. Higher and more lateral
40. LAO (or RPO if the patient cannot lie supine)
41. A. 40°
    B. 15°
42. Erect or right lateral decubitus
43. Right lateral decubitus (PA)
44. B. 5 to 10 mrad
45. 1 to 2 in (2.5 to 5 cm)

Review Exercise C: Problem Solving for Technical and Positioning Errors
1. Center the CR lower and more mid-line for an asthenic patient. Also, using a 14 × 17 inch (35 × 43 cm) image receptor for the scout, instead of a 10 × 12 inch (24 × 30 cm), will provide greater coverage of the abdomen.
2. Lower the kV to the 70 to 76 range.
3. Increase body rotation to project the gallbladder away from the spine.
4. Request that the patient be rotated into a 15° to 25° RPO position or place the cassette and grid in a crosswise alignment and angle the CR 15° to 25° in a mediolateral direction.
5. Ultrasound of the gallbladder. It does not require any contrast media.
6. Percutaneous transhepatic cholangiogram (PTC) (The PTC may also be preceded by an ultrasound study.)
7. A nuclear medicine hepatobiliary or HIDA scan can provide information on the anatomy and function of the gallbladder.
8. ERCP
9. Sonography or nuclear medicine HIDA scan
10. Sonography or computed tomography

16

SELF-TEST

My Score = _____ %

Directions: This self-test should be taken only after completing all of the readings, review exercises, and laboratory activities for a particular section. The purpose of this test is not only to provide a good learning exercise but also to serve as a good indicator of what your final evaluation exam will be. It is strongly suggested that if you do not get at least a 90% to 95% grade on each self-test, you review those areas in which you missed questions before going to your instructor for the final evaluation exam for this chapter. (There are 70 questions or blanks—each is worth 1.4 points.)

1. The gallbladder is located in the _____ margin of the liver.

   A. Anterior inferior   C. Mid aspect

   B. Posterior superior   D. Anterior superior

2. Which one of the following is **not** a major lobe of the liver?

   A. Caudate   C. Inferior

   B. Quadrate   D. Left

3. In which quadrant is the liver located in the average patient?

   A. Right lower quadrant   C. Left upper quadrant

   B. Left lower quadrant   D. Right upper quadrant

4. What is the name of the soft-tissue structure that divides the liver into left and right lobes?

   _____

5. What is the primary function of bile? _____

6. Which duct is formed by the union of the left and right hepatic ducts? _____

7. What is the average capacity of the gallbladder? _____

8. Which chemical process leads to concentration of bile within the gallbladder? _____

9. Which hormone leads to contraction of the gallbladder to release bile? _____

10. Which duct carries bile from the cystic duct to the duodenum? _____

11.   Match each of the following biliary structures to its correct description or definition:

      _____   1.   Pancreatic duct   A.   Series of mucosal folds in cystic duct

      _____   2.   Fundus   B.   A protrusion into the duodenum

      _____   3.   Hepatopancreatic ampulla   C.   Middle aspect of gallbladder

      _____   4.   Spiral valve   D.   Duct connected directly to gallbladder

      _____   5.   Hepatopancreatic sphincter   E.   Narrowest portion of gallbladder

      _____   6.   Duodenal papilla   F.   Broadest portion of gallbladder

      _____   7.   Cystic duct   G.   Enlarged chamber in distal aspect of common bile duct

      _____   8.   Neck   H.   Duct of Wirsung

      _____   9.   Body   I.   Circular muscle

12.   A.   Which general body position will encourage drainage of bile/contrast media from the gallbladder?

      _____

      B.   Why? _____

13.   Identify the labeled parts and/or structures on the radiograph of an OCG (Fig. 16-3) and of biliary ducts from an operative cholangiogram procedure (Fig. 16-4).

      Fig. 16-3:

      A. _____

      B. _____

      C. _____

      D. _____

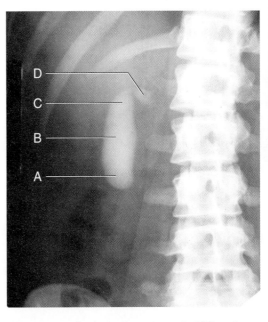

Fig. 16-3. Radiograph of an OCG and of biliary ducts.

16

Fig. 16-4:

E. _____

F. _____

G. _____

H. _____

I. _____

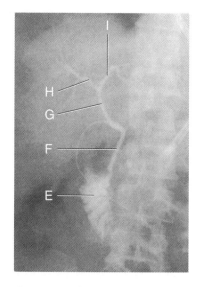

Fig. 16-4. Radiograph of an operative cholangiogram procedure.

14. Match each of the following terms with its corresponding definition or description.

_____	1. Cysto-	A.	Radiographic study of gallbladder and biliary ducts
_____	2. Chole-	B.	Radiographic study of gallbladder
_____	3. Cholecystocholangiogram	C.	Radiographic study of biliary ducts
_____	4. Cholecystogram	D.	Condition of having gallstones
_____	5. Cholangiogram	E.	Inflammation of gallbladder
_____	6. Cholecystopaque	F.	Oral contrast media for gallbladder
_____	7. Cholecystitis	G.	OCG
_____	8. Oral cholecystogram	H.	Denotes sac or bladder
_____	9. Cholelithiasis	I.	Denotes bile

15. True/False: Drugs have been developed that will dissolve gallstones and may avoid the need to have surgery in select cases.

16. True/False: Gallbladders with acute cholecystitis rarely become radiopaque during an OCG.

17. Match each of the following pathologic indications with its correct definition or description:

_____ 1. Biliary stenosis   A. Emulsion of biliary stones

_____ 2. Congenital anomalies   B. May be caused by bacterial infection or ischemia of the gallbladder

_____ 3. Chronic cholecystitis   C. Narrowing of one of the biliary ducts

_____ 4. Choledocholithiasis   D. Although benign, they may affect production, storage, or release of bile

_____ 5. Acute cholecystitis   E. Signs may include calcification of the gallbladder wall

_____ 6. Milk calcium bile   F. Approximately 80% of patients with this condition have gallstones

_____ 7. Carcinoma of gallbladder   G. Stones in the biliary ducts

18. How long should a patient remain NPO before an OCG? _____

19. How far in advance should the oral contrast medium be taken for an OCG? _____

20. Which kV range is ideal for an OCG? _____

21. True/False: Ultrasound of the gallbladder requires that the patient be NPO for at least 8 hours before the study.

22. True/False: Ultrasound of the gallbladder is considered a noninvasive procedure.

23. How is the contrast medium instilled into the biliary ducts during an ERCP?

_____

24. Which of the following is one of the more common risks associated with a PTC?
    A. Pancreatitis   C. Biliary stenosis
    B. Pneumothorax   D. GI bleed

25. What does the acronym ERCP actually mean? _____

26. Other than a radiologist, what type of physician often performs ERCPs? _____

27. What is the most common clinical reason for performing a T-tube cholangiogram?

_____

28. Which one of the following is a pathologic indication for a percutaneous transhepatic cholangiogram (PTC)?
    A. Chronic cholecystitis   C. Neoplasm of the gallbladder
    B. Obstructive jaundice   D. Cholelithiasis

29. What type of needle is most often used for a PTC?
    A. 6-inch spinal needle   C. 18-gauge angiocath
    B. 18-gauge butterfly   D. Skinny, or Chiba, needle

16

30. Match the following by indicating whether each procedure is performed in the operating room by a **surgeon (S)** or performed in the radiology department by a **radiologist (R).**

    _____   A.   T-tube cholangiogram   S.   In operating room by a surgeon

    _____   B.   Operative cholangiogram   R.   In radiology department by a radiologist

    _____   C.   Percutaneous transhepatic cholangiogram

31. True/False: An ERCP can be considered both a diagnostic and therapeutic procedure.

32. True/False: A percutaneous transhepatic cholangiogram (PTC) is generally performed in the radiology department and involves placing a needle through the liver directly into a biliary duct.

33. True/False: A pediatric patient with hemolytic anemia may develop gallstones.

34. True/False: A HIDA scan is a special MRI study of the liver using a contrast agent.

35. True/False: CT is an excellent imaging modality for demonstrating tumors of the liver, gallbladder, or pancreas.

36. Which ionization chamber (right, left, or center) needs to be activated for an LAO projection of the gallbladder?

    _____

37. **Situation:** An asthenic patient comes to the radiology department for an OCG. The technologist is unsure where to center for the PA scout image. Where should the CR be centered for this patient?

    _____

16

38. **Situation:** A radiograph of an LAO projection reveals that the gallbladder is superimposed over the spine. What modification is needed during the repeat exposure to avoid this problem?

    _____

39. Why is the erect gallbladder projection preferred as a PA rather than an AP projection?

    _____

40. **Situation:** During an OCG, the radiologist believes that stones may be present in the gallbladder. She requests that the technologist provide a projection to stratify any possible stones. Which two projections may accomplish this goal?

    _____

41. **Situation:** A patient scheduled for an OCG complains that she cannot lie prone or on her right side because of recent surgery. Which position could be performed to ensure that the gallbladder will not be superimposed over the spine?

    _____

42. **Situation:** A patient with a history of possible gallstones is scheduled for an OCG. During the patient interview, she states that she had a piece of bacon before coming into the hospital. When the scout image is taken, the gallbladder is not visualized. What other imaging options can the radiologist order to determine whether there are gallbladder stones?

    _____

43. Which one of the following studies is considered an invasive procedure?

    A.   OCG   C.   Sonography of the gallbladder

    B.   CT of the gallbladder   D.   PTC

Urinary System

After you have successfully completed the activities in this chapter, you will be able to:

_____ 1. Identify the location and pertinent anatomy of the urinary system to include the adrenal glands.

_____ 2. Identify specific structures of the macroscopic and microscopic anatomy and physiology of the kidney.

_____ 3. Identify the orientation of the kidneys, ureters, and urinary bladder with respect to the peritoneum and other structures of the abdomen.

_____ 4. List the primary functions of the urinary system.

_____ 5. Describe the spatial relationship between the male and female reproductive system and the urinary system.

_____ 6. On drawings and radiographs, identify specific anatomy of the urinary system.

_____ 7. Identify key lab values and drug concerns that must be verified prior to intravenous injections of contrast media.

_____ 8. Identify characteristics specific to either ionic or nonionic contrast media.

_____ 9. Describe the four categories of contrast media reactions and the symptoms specific to each type of reaction.

_____ 10. Differentiate between mild, moderate, and severe levels of contrast media reactions and from side effects to iodinated contrast media.

_____ 11. Identify the steps and safety measures to be observed during a venipuncture procedure.

_____ 12. List safety measures to be followed before and during the injection of an iodinated contrast media.

_____ 13. Define specific urinary pathologic terminology and indicators.

_____ 14. Match specific types of urinary pathology to the correct radiographic appearances and signs.

_____ 15. List the purpose, contraindications, and ten high-risk patient conditions for intravenous urography.

_____ 16. Identify two methods used to enhance pelvicalyceal filling during intravenous urography and contraindications for their use.

_____ 17. Explain the difference between a nephrogram and a nephrotomogram.

_____ 18. Identify specific aspects related to the retrograde urogram and how this procedure differs from an intravenous urogram (IVU).

_____ 19. Identify specific aspects related to the retrograde cystogram.

_____ 20. Identify specific aspects related to the retrograde urethrogram.

_____ 21. List specific information related to the basic and special projections for excretory urography, retrograde urography, cystography, urethrography, and voiding cystourethrography to include size and type of image receptor (IR), central ray location, direction and angulation of central ray, and anatomy best visualized.

_____ 22. Identify the patient dose ranges for skin, midline, and gonads for specific urinary system projections.

_____ 23. Given various hypothetical situations, identify the correct modification of a position and/or exposure factors to improve the radiographic image.

Positioning and Radiographic Critique

_____ 1. Using a peer, position for basic and special projections for an intravenous urogram procedure.

_____ 2. Critique and evaluate urinary study radiographs based on the four divisions of radiographic criteria: (1) structures shown, (2) position, (3) collimation and CR, and (4) exposure criteria.

_____ 3. Distinguish between acceptable and unacceptable urinary study radiographs based on exposure factors, motion, collimation, positioning, or other errors.

Learning Exercises

The following review exercises should be completed only after careful study of the associated pages in the textbook as indicated by each exercise. Answers to each review exercise are given at the end of the review exercises.

Part I: Radiographic Anatomy

REVIEW EXERCISE A: Radiographic Anatomy of the Urinary System (see textbook pp. 544-550)

1. The kidneys and ureters are located in the _____ space.

    A. Intraperitoneal   C. Extraperitoneal

    B. Infraperitoneal   D. Retroperitoneal

2. The _____ glands are located directly superior to the kidneys.

3. Which structures create a 20° angle between the upper pole and lower pole of the kidney?_____

4. What is the specific name for the mass of fat that surrounds each kidney? _____

5. What degree of rotation from supine is required to place the kidneys parallel to the IR? _____

6. Which two bony landmarks can be palpated to locate the kidneys?_____

7. Which term describes an abnormal drop of the kidneys when the patient is placed erect? _____

8. List the three functions of the urinary system:

    A. _____

    B. _____

    C. _____

9. A buildup of nitrogenous waste in the blood is called:

    A. Hemotoxicity   C. Sepsis

    B. Uremia   D. Renotoxicity

10. The longitudinal fissure found along the central medial border of the kidney is called the _____ .

11. The peripheral or outer portion of the kidney is called the _____ .

12. The term that describes the total functioning portion of the kidney is _____ .

13. The microscopic function and structural unit of the kidney is the _____ .

14. Which structure of the medulla is made up of a collection of tubules that drain into the minor calyx?

    _____

15. What is another (older) name for the glomerular capsule? _____

16. True/False: The glomerular capsule and proximal and distal convoluted tubules are located in the medulla of the kidney.

17. True/False: The efferent arterioles carry blood to the glomeruli.

18. Identify the renal structures labeled on Fig. 17-1:

    A. _____

    B. _____

    C. _____

    D. _____

    E. _____

    F. _____

    G. _____

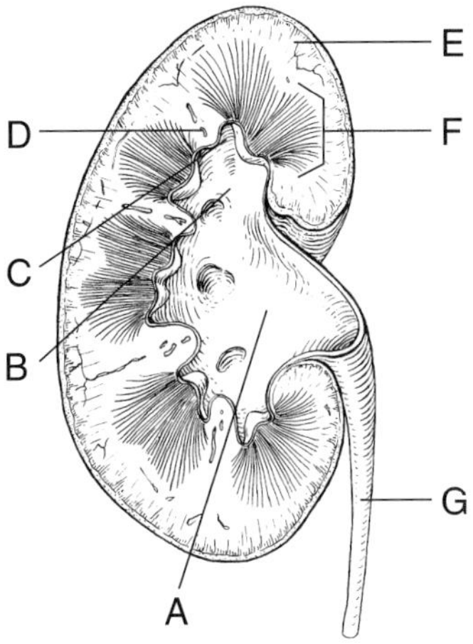

Fig. 17-1. Cross-section of a kidney.

19. Identify the structures making up a nephron and collecting duct (Fig. 17-2). For each structure, indicate with a check mark whether it is located in the cortex or medulla portion of the kidney.

STRUCTURE	CORTEX	MEDULLA
A. _____	_____	_____
B. _____	_____	_____
C. _____	_____	_____
D. _____	_____	_____
E. _____	_____	_____
F. _____	_____	_____
G. _____	_____	_____
H. _____	_____	_____
I. _____	_____	_____

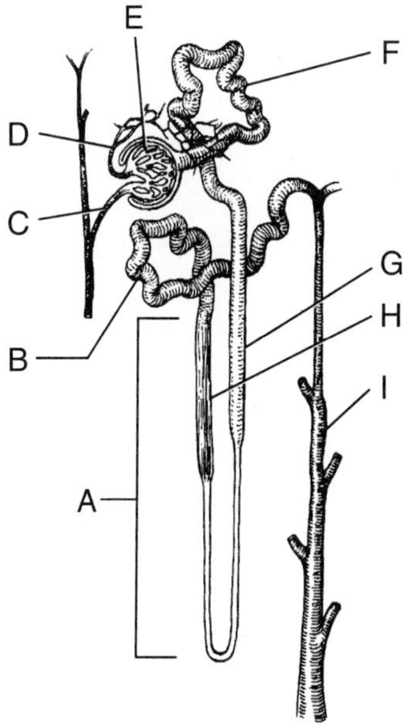

Fig. 17-2. Structures of a nephron and collecting duct.

20. Which two processes move urine through the ureters to the bladder?

    A. _____   B. _____

21. Which one of the following structures is located most anterior as compared with the others?

    A. Proximal ureters   C. Urinary bladder

    B. Kidneys   D. Suprarenal glands

22. What is the name of the junction found between the distal ureters and urinary bladder? _____

23. What is the name of the inner, posterior region of the bladder formed by the two ureters entering and the urethra exiting?

    _____

24. What is the name of the small gland found just inferior to the male bladder? _____

25. The total capacity for the average adult bladder is:

    A. 100 to 200 ml   C. 350 to 500 ml

    B. 200 to 300 ml   D. 500 to 700 ml

26. Which one of the following structures is considered to be most posterior?

    A. Ovaries   C. Vagina

    B. Urethra   D. Kidneys

27. Identify the urinary structures labeled on Fig. 17-3:

    A. _____

    B. _____

    C. _____

    D. _____

    E. _____

    F. _____

    G. _____

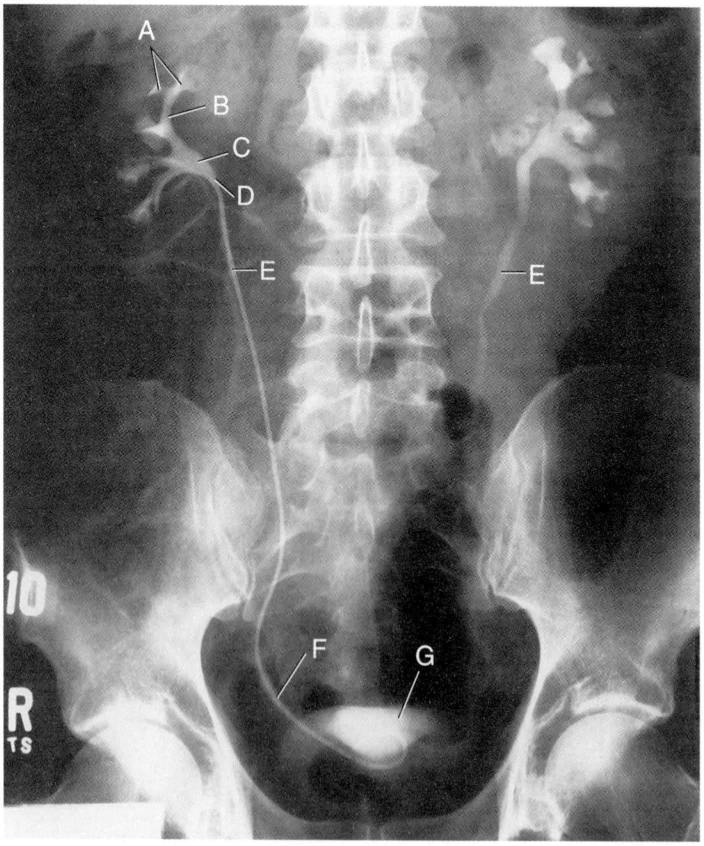

Fig. 17-3. AP retrograde pyelogram radiograph.

Part II: Radiographic Positioning, Contrast Media, and Pathology

REVIEW EXERCISE B: Venipuncture (see textbook pp. 551-554)

1. Intravenous contrast media may be administered by either:

   A. _____

   B. _____

2. True/False: The patient (or legal guardian) must sign an informed consent form before a venipuncture procedure is performed on a pediatric patient.

3. For most IVUs, veins in the _____ are recommended for venipuncture.

   A. Iliac fossa   C. Axillary fossa

   B. Anterior, carpal region   D. Antecubital fossa

4. The most common size of needle used for bolus injections of contrast media is:

   A. 23 to 25 gauge   C. 18 to 20 gauge

   B. 14 to 16 gauge   D. 28 gauge

5. The two most common types of needles used for bolus injection of contrast media are _____

   and _____ .

6. In the correct order, list the eight steps followed during a venipuncture procedure as listed and described in the textbook (pp. 553-554):

   A. _____

   B. _____

   C. _____

   D. _____

   E. _____

   F. _____

   G. _____

   H. _____

7. True/False: The bevel of the needle needs to be facing downward during the actual puncture into a vein.

8. True/False: If extravasation occurs during the puncture, the technologist should slightly retract the needle and then push it forward again.

9. True/False: If unsuccessful during the initial puncture, a new needle should be used during the second attempt.

10. True/False: The radiologist is responsible for documenting all aspects of the venipuncture procedure in the patient's chart.

17

REVIEW EXERCISE C: Contrast Media and Urography (see textbook pp. 555-559)

1. The two major types of iodinated contrast media used for urography are ionic and nonionic. Indicate whether each of the following characteristics applies to ionic (I) or nonionic (N) contrast media:

    _____ A. Uses a parent compound of a benzoic acid

    _____ B. Will not significantly increase the osmolality of the blood plasma

    _____ D. Incorporates sodium or meglumine to increase solubility of the contrast media

    _____ D. Creates a hypertonic condition in the blood plasma

    _____ E. Is more expensive

    _____ F. Produces less severe reactions

    _____ G. Is a near-isotonic solution

    _____ H. Poses a greater risk for disrupting homeostasis

    _____ I. Uses a parent compound of an amide or glucose group

    _____ J. May increase the severity of side effects

2. Which one of the following compounds is a common **anion** found in ionic contrast media?

    A. Diatrizoate or iothalamate   C. Benzoic acid

    B. Sodium or meglumine   D. None of the above

3. Any disruption in the physiological functions of the body that may lead to a contrast media reaction is the basis for the:

    A. Homeostasis theory   C. Vasovagal theory

    B. Anaphylactoid theory   D. Chemotoxic theory

4. The normal creatinine level for an adult should range between _____ .

5. Normal BUN levels for an adult should range between _____ .

6. A. Glucophage is a drug that is taken for the management of _____ .

    B. The American College of Radiology recommends that Glucophage be withheld for _____

    hours before a contrast media procedure and not taken for _____ hours following a contrast media procedure.

7. List ten contraindications that may prevent a patient from having a contrast media procedure performed.

    A. _____   F. _____

    B. _____   G _____

    C. _____   H. _____

    D. _____   I. _____

    E. _____   J. _____

8. List the four types or categories of contrast media reactions:

    A. _____

    B. _____

    C. _____

    D. _____

9. Which type of reaction is a true allergic response to iodinated contrast media? _____

10. Which type of reaction is due to the stimulation of the vagus nerve by introduction of contrast media, which causes

    heart rate and blood pressure to fall? _____

11. True/False: Vasovagal reactions are not considered to be life-threatening.

12. True/False: Acute renal failure may occur 48 hours following an iodinated contrast media procedure.

13. Matching: Match the following symptoms to the correct type of contrast media reaction (more than one symptom
    may apply to a type of reaction):

    _____ A. Brachycardia (< 50 beats/minute)   1. Vasomotor effect

    _____ B. Tachycardia (> 100 beats/minute)   2. Anaphylactic reaction

    _____ C. Angioedema   3. Vasovagal reaction

    _____ D. Syncope   4. Acute renal failure

    _____ E. Hypotension (systolic blood pressure < 80 mm Hg)

    _____ F. Anuria

    _____ G. Laryngospasm

    _____ H. Lightheadedness

    _____ I. No detectable pulse

14. True/False: Mild-level contrast media reactions are usually self-limiting and do not require medication.

15. True/False: Urticaria is the formal term for excessive vomiting.

16. The leakage of contrast media from a vessel into the surrounding soft tissues is called _____ .

17. A reaction based on fear or anxiety is called _____ .

18. An expected outcome to the introduction of contrast media is described as a _____ .

17

19. Matching: For each of the following symptoms, identify the severity (1-4) of contrast media reactions (may be used more than once):

    _____ A. Convulsions   1. Side effect

    _____ B. Metallic taste   2. Mild level

    _____ C. Cyanosis   3. Moderate level

    _____ D. Giant hives   4. Severe level

    _____ E. Itching

    _____ F. Vasomotor response

    _____ G. Temporary hot flash

    _____ H. Difficulty in breathing

    _____ I. Laryngeal spasm

    _____ J. Extravasation

    _____ K. Excessive urticaria

20. What should the technologist do first when a patient is experiencing either a moderate or a severe level contrast media reaction? _____

21. What is the primary purpose of the premedication protocol prior to an iodinated contrast media procedure?

_____

22. Which of the following drugs is often given to the patient as part of the premedication protocol?
   A. Epinephrine   C. Combination of Benadryl and prednisone
   B. Valium   D. Lasix

REVIEW EXERCISE D: Radiographic Procedures and Pathologic Terms and Indications (see textbook pp. 560-570)

1. A. Why is the term *IVP* incorrect in describing a radiographic examination of the kidneys, ureters, and bladder following intravenous injection of contrast media?

   _____

   B. What is the correct term and correct abbreviation for the exam described in question 1?

   _____

2. Which specific aspect of the kidney is visualized during an IVU? _____

3. Which one of the following conditions is a common pathologic indication for an IVU?
   A. Sickle cell anemia   C. Hematuria
   B. Multiple myeloma   D. Anuria

17

4. Which one of the following conditions is described as a rare tumor of the kidney?

    A. Pheochromocytoma   C. Melanoma

    B. Multiple myeloma   D. Renal cell carcinoma

5. Matching: Match each of the following urinary pathologic terms to its correct definition:

    _____ A. Pneumouria   1. Passage of large volume of urine

    _____ B. Urinary reflux   2. Presence of glucose in urine

    _____ C. Uremia   3. Excess urea and creatinine in the blood

    _____ D. Anuria   4. Diminished amount of urine being excreted

    _____ E. Polyuria   5. Presence of gas in urine

    _____ F. Micturition   6. Indicated by presence of uremia, oliguria, or anuria

    _____ G. Retention   7. Constant or frequent involuntary passage of urine

    _____ H. Oliguria   8. Backward return flow of urine

    _____ I. Glucosuria   9. Absence of a functioning kidney

    _____ J. Urinary incontinence   10. Complete cessation of urinary secretion

    _____ K. Renal agenesis   11. Act of voiding

    _____ L. Acute renal failure   12. Inability to void

6. Match each of the following descriptions to the correct pathologic indication:

    _____ A. Age-associated enlargement of the   1. Vesicorectal fistula
                 prostate gland
                                                            2. Renal hypertension
    _____ B. Fusion of the kidney during the
                 development of the fetus   3. Ectopic kidney

    _____ C. Inflammation of the capillary loops   4. Horseshoe kidney
                 of the glomeruli of the kidneys
                                                            5. Staghorn calculus
    _____ D. Artificial opening between
                 the urinary bladder and aspects of the   6. Polycystic kidney disease
                 large intestine
                                                            7. Benign prostatic hyperplasia
    _____ E. A large stone that grows and completely
                 fills the renal pelvis   8. Glomerulonephritis

    _____ F. Increased blood pressure to the kidneys
                 due to atherosclerosis

    _____ G. Normal kidney that fails to ascend
                 into the abdomen but remains in the pelvis

    _____ H. Multiple cysts in one or both kidneys

17

7. Match each of the following radiographic appearances to the correct pathologic indication:

    _____ A. Rapid excretion of contrast media   1. Malrotation

    _____ B. Mucosal changes within bladder   2. Vesicorectal fistula

    _____ C. Bilateral, small kidneys with blunted calyces   3. Renal cell carcinoma

    _____ D. Irregular appearance of renal parenchyma or collecting system   4. BPH

    _____ E. Signs of abnormal fluid collections   5. Renal hypertension

    _____ F. Abnormal rotation of the kidney   6. Renal calculi

    _____ G. Elevated or indented floor of bladder   7. Cystitis

    _____ H. Signs of obstruction of urinary system   8. Chronic Bright disease

8. A condition characterized by regions or areas of subcutaneous swelling due to allergic reaction to foods or drugs is termed _____.

9. Contraction of the muscles within the walls of the bronchi and bronchioles, producing a restriction of air passing through them, is a condition called _____.

10. Loss of consciousness due to reduced cerebral blood flow is termed _____.

11. A trademark for a diuretic drug used in treatment of renal disease is _____.

12. An eruption of wheals (hives) often due to a hypersensitivity to food or drugs is a condition termed

_____.

13. True/False: If an IVU and barium enema are both scheduled, the IVU should always be performed first.

14. True/False: The patient should void before an IVU to prevent possible rupture of the bladder if compression is applied.

15. What is the primary purpose of ureteric compression? _____

16. List the six conditions that could contraindicate the use of ureteric compression:

    A. _____   D. _____

    B. _____   E. _____

    C. _____   F. _____

17. When does the timing for an IVU exam start? _____

18. List the basic five-step imaging sequence for a routine IVU:

    A. _____   D. _____

    B. _____   E. _____

    C. _____

19. What is the primary difference between a standard and a hypertensive IVU?

_____

20. In which department are most retrograde urograms performed? _____

21. True/False: A retrograde urogram examines the anatomy and function of the pelvicalyceal system.

22. True/False: The Brodney clamp is used for male and female retrograde cystourethrograms.

23. Which of the following involves a direct introduction of the contrast media into the structure being studied?

    A. Retrograde urogram   C. Retrograde urethrogram

    B. Retrograde cystogram   D. All of the above

24. Which of the following alternative imaging modalities is NOT being used to diagnose renal calculi?

    A. Nuclear medicine   C. Magnetic resonance imaging

    B. Sonography   D. Computed tomography

25. True/False: Urinary studies on pediatric patients should be scheduled early in the morning to minimize the risk for dehydration.

26. True/False: Nuclear medicine is highly effective in demonstrating signs of vesicoureteral reflux.

27. True/False: The number of retrograde urography procedures for urethral calculi has been reduced as a result of the increased use of CT.

28. Who should the technologist contact if he or she has difficulty placing the needle into the vein of a pediatric patient

    during IVU? _____

REVIEW EXERCISE E: Radiographic Positioning of the Urinary System (see textbook pp. 571-578)

1. What are the four reasons a scout projection is taken prior to the injection of contrast media for an IVU?

    A. _____   C. _____

    B. _____   D. _____

2. What kV range is recommended for an IVU? _____

3. Which ionization chambers should be activated for an AP scout projection? _____

4. True/False: Both the female midline dose and the female gonadal dose for an average unshielded AP projection for an IVU are in the 100 to 200 mrad range.

5. True/False: Male and female patients should have the gonads shielded for an AP scout projection.

6. True/False: Tomograms taken during an IVU with an exposure angle of 10° or less are called _zonography._

7. How many tomograms (zonograms) are usually produced during a typical IVU? _____

8. At what stage of an IVU is the renal parenchyma best seen?

    A. 5 minutes following injection   C. After the postvoid projection

    B. 10 minutes following injection   D. Within 1 minute following injection

17

9.   Where is the CR centered for a nephrotomogram?

    A.   At xiphoid process   C.   At iliac crest

    B.   Midway between xiphoid process and iliac crest   D.   At axillary costal margin

10.   Which specific position, taken during an IVU, will place the left kidney parallel to the IR? _____

11.   How much obliquity is required for the LPO/RPO projections taken during an IVU? _____

12.   Which position will best demonstrate possible nephroptosis? _____

13.   How will an enlarged prostate gland appear on a postvoid radiograph taken during an IVU?

    _____

14.   Where should the pneumatic paddle be placed for the ureteric compression phase of an IVU?

    _____

15.   What can be done to enhance filling of the calyces of the kidney if ureteric compression is contraindicated?

    _____

16.   What specific anatomy is examined during a retrograde ureterogram?

    A.   Primarily the ureters   C.   Entire urinary system

    B.   Primarily the renal pelvis and calyces   D.   Urinary bladder

17.   A retrograde pyelogram is primarily a nonfunctional study of the _____ .

18.   What CR angle is used for the AP projection taken during a cystogram?

    A.   20° to 25° caudad   C.   10° to 15° caudad

    B.   5° to 10° cephalad   D.   30° to 40° caudad

19.   True/False: For a lateral cystogram, both the male and female dose are in the 100 (±50) mrad range.

20.   Which specific position is recommended for a male patient during a voiding cystourethrogram? _____

REVIEW EXERCISE F: Problem Solving for Technical and Positioning Errors (see textbook pp. 561-578)

1.   **Situation:** A radiograph of an AP scout projection of the abdomen, taken during an IVU, reveals that the symphysis pubis is cut off slightly. The patient is too large to include the entire abdomen on a 35 × 43 cm (14 × 17 inch) IR. What should the technologist do in this situation?

    _____

    _____

17

2. **Situation:** A nephrogram is ordered as part of an IVU study. When the nephrogram image is processed, there is a minimal amount of contrast media within the renal parenchyma and the calyces are beginning to fill with contrast media. What specific problem led to this radiographic outcome?

_____

_____

3. **Situation:** A 45° RPO radiograph taken during an IVU reveals that the left kidney is foreshortened. What modification is needed to improve this image during the repeat exposure?

_____

_____

4. **Situation:** An AP projection taken during the compression phase of an IVU reveals that the majority of the contrast media has left the collecting system of the kidneys. The technologist placed the pneumatic paddles near the umbilicus and ensured that they were inflated. What can the technologist do to ensure better retention of contrast media in the collecting system during the compression phase of future IVUs?

_____

_____

5. **Situation:** An AP projection radiograph taken during a cystogram reveals that the floor of the bladder is superimposed over the symphysis pubis. What can the technologist do to correct this problem during the repeat exposure?

_____

_____

6. **Situation:** A patient comes to the radiology department for an IVU. While taking the clinical history, the technologist learns the patient has renal hypertension. How must the technologist modify the IVU imaging sequence to accommodate this patient's condition?

_____

_____

7. **Situation:** A patient comes to the radiology department for an IVU. The AP scout reveals an abnormal density near the lumbar spine that the radiologist suspects is an abdominal aortic aneurysm. What should the technologist do about the ureteric compression phase of the study that is part of the procedure protocol?

_____

_____

17

8. **Situation:** A patient comes to the radiology department for an IVU. The patient history indicates that he may have an enlarged prostate gland. Which projection will best demonstrate this condition?

_____

_____

9. **Situation:** A patient with a history of bladder calculi comes to the radiology department. A retrograde cystogram has been ordered. During the interview, the patient reports that he had a severe reaction to contrast media in the past. What other imaging modality(ies) can be performed to best diagnose this condition?

_____

10. **Situation:** The same patient described in question 9 may also have calculi in the kidney. What is the preferred imaging modality for this situation when iodinated contrast media cannot be used?

_____

11. **Situation:** A patient comes to the radiology department for an IVU. As the patient's clinical history is being reviewed, it is discovered that he is diabetic. What additional question(s) should the patient be asked during the interview prior to the procedure?

_____

_____

12. **Situation:** During an IVU, the patient complains of a metallic taste and has a sudden urge to urinate. What action should the technologist take?

_____

_____

Part III: Laboratory Exercises (see textbook pp. 571-578)

Although it is impossible to duplicate many aspects of urinary studies on a phantom in the lab, evaluation of actual radiographs and physical positioning is possible. You can get experience in positioning and radiographic evaluation of these projections by performing exercises using radiographic phantoms and practicing on other students (although you will not be taking actual exposures). Technologists must learn the positioning routine, room setup, and fluoroscopy procedure for their particular facility.

LABORATORY EXERCISE A: Radiographic Evaluation

1. Using actual radiographs of IVU, cystogram, and retrograde urogram procedures provided by your instructor, evaluate each position for the following points (check off when completed):

   _____ Evaluate the completeness of the study. (Are all pertinent anatomic structures included on the radiograph?)

   _____ Evaluate for positioning or centering errors (e.g., rotation, off centering)

   _____ Evaluate for correct exposure factors and possible motion. (Is the contrast medium properly penetrated?)

   _____ Determine whether patient rotation is correct for specific positions.

   _____ Determine whether markers and an acceptable degree of collimation and/or area shielding are visible on the images.

17

LABORATORY EXERCISE B: Physical Positioning

On another person, simulate performing all basic and special projections of the IVU as follows. Include the six steps listed below and described in the textbook. (Check off each when completed satisfactorily.)

Step 1. Appropriate size and type of image receptor with correct markers
Step 2. Correct CR placement and centering of part to CR and/or image receptor
Step 3. Accurate collimation
Step 4. Area shielding of patient where advisable
Step 5. Use of proper immobilizing devices when needed
Step 6. Approximate correct exposure factors, breathing instructions where applicable, and "making" exposure

PROJECTIONS	*STEP 1*	*STEP 2*	*STEP 3*	*STEP 4*	*STEP 5*	*STEP 6*
• AP scout	____	____	____	____	____	____
• LPO and RPO	____	____	____	____	____	____
• AP cystogram	____	____	____	____	____	____
• Lateral cystogram	____	____	____	____	____	____

17

Answers to Review Exercises

Review Exercise A: Radiographic Anatomy of the Urinary System

1. D. Retroperitoneal
2. Suprarenal glands
3. Psoas muscles
4. Perirenal fat, or adipose capsule
5. 30°
6. Xiphoid process and iliac crest
7. Nephroptosis
8. A. Remove nitrogenous waste
   B. Regulate water levels
   C. Regulate acid-base balance
9. B. Uremia
10. Hilum
11. Cortex
12. Renal parenchyma
13. Nephron
14. Renal pyramids
15. Bowman's capsule
16. False (located in the cortex)
17. False (afferent)
18. A. Renal pelvis
   B. Major calyx
   C. Minor calyx
   D. Renal sinuses
   E. Cortex
   F. Medulla
   G. Ureter
19. A. Loop of Henle, medulla
   B. Distal convoluted tubule, cortex
   C. Afferent arteriole, cortex
   D. Efferent arteriole, cortex
   E. Glomerular capsule, cortex
   F. Proximal convoluted tubule, cortex
   G. Descending limb, medulla
   H. Ascending limb, medulla
   I. Collecting tubule, medulla
20. A. Peristalsis
   B. Gravity
21. C. Urinary bladder
22. Ureterovesical junction
23. Trigone
24. Prostate gland
25. C. 350 to 500 ml
26. D. Kidneys
27. A. Minor calyces
   B. Major calyces
   C. Renal pelvis
   D. Ureteropelvic junction (UPJ)
   E. Proximal ureter
   F. Distal ureter
   G. Urinary bladder

Review Exercise B: Venipuncture

1. A. Bolus injection
   B. Drip infusion
2. True
3. D. Antecubital fossa
4. C. 18 to 20 gauge
5. Butterfly and over-the-needle catheter
6. A. Wash hands and put on gloves
   B. Select site and apply tourniquet
   C. Confirm puncture site and cleanse
   D. Initiate puncture
   E. Confirm entry and secure needle
   F. Prepare for Injection
   G. Proceed with injection
   H. Needle or catheter
7. False (facing upward)
8. False (Needle should be withdrawn and pressure applied.)
9. True
10. False (Technologist or the person performing the venipuncture is responsible.)

Review Exercise C: Contrast Media and Urography

1. A. I
   B. N
   C. I
   D. I
   E. N
   F. N
   G. N
   H. I
   I. N
   J. I
2. A. Diatrizoate or iothalamate
3. D. Chemotoxic theory
4. 0.6 to 1.5 mg/dl
5. 8 to 25 mg/100 ml
6. A. Diabetes mellitus
   B. 48 hours, 48 hours
7. A. Hypersensitivity to iodinated contrast media
   B. Anuria
   C. Multiple myeloma
   D. Diabetes mellitus
   E. Severe hepatic or renal disease
   F. Congestive heart failure
   G. Pheochromocytoma
   H. Sickle cell anemia
   I. Patients taking Glucophage
   J. Renal failure, acute or chronic
8. A. Vasomotor effect
   B. Anaphylactic reaction
   C. Vasovagal reaction
   D. Acute renal failure
9. Anaphylactic reaction
10. Vasovagal reaction
11. False
12. True
13. A. 3
   B. 2
   C. 2

D. 1
E. 3
F. 4
G. 2
H. 1
I. 3
14. True
15. False (the term for hives)
16. Extravasation
17. Vasomotor effect
18. Side effect
19. A. 4
   B. 1
   C. 4
   D. 3
   E. 2
   F. 2
   G. 1
   H. 4
   I. 4
   J. 2
   K. 3
20. Call for medical assistance
21. To reduce the risk for contrast media reactions
22. C. Combination of Benadryl and prednisone

Review Exercise D: Radiographic Procedures and Pathologic Terms and Indications

1. A. An IVP (intravenous pyelogram) is a study of the renal pelvis (hence, *pyelo-*).
   B. Intravenous urogram (IVU)
2. The collecting system of the kidney
3. C. Hematuria
4. A. Pheochromocytoma
5. A. 5
   B. 8
   C. 3
   D. 10
   E. 1
   F. 11
   G. 12
   H. 4
   I. 2
   J. 7
   K. 9
   L. 6
6. A. 7
   B. 4
   C. 8
   D. 1
   E. 5
   F. 2
   G. 3
   H. 6

17

7. A. 5
   B. 7
   C. 8
   D. 3
   E. 2
   F. 1
   G. 4
   H. 6
8. Angioedema
9. Bronchospasm
10. Syncope
11. Lasix
12. Urticaria
13. True
14. True
15. To enhance filling of the pelvica-
    lyceal system with contrast
    media
16. A. Possible ureteric stones
    B. Abdominal mass
    C. Abdominal aortic aneurysm
    D. Recent abdominal surgery
    E. Severe abdominal pain
    F. Acute abdominal trauma
17. At start of injection of contrast
    media
18. A. 1-minute nephrogram or nephro-
       tomography
    B. 5-minute full KUB
    C. 15-minute full KUB
    D. 20-minute posterior R and L
       oblique positions
    E. Postvoid (prone PA or erect AP)
19. A hypertensive IVU requires a
    shorter span of time between pro-
    jections.
20. In surgery
21. False (nonfunctional exam)
22. False (used for males only)
23. D. All of the above
24. C. Magnetic resonance imaging
25. True
26. True
27. True
28. A phlebotomist or physician

Review Exercise E: Radiographic Positioning of the Urinary System

1. A. Verify patient preparation
   B. Determine whether exposure fac-
      tors are acceptable
   C. Verify positioning
   D. Detect any abnormal calcifications
2. 70 to 75 kV
3. Upper right and left ionization
   chambers
4. False (in the 30 to 50 mrad range)
5. False (not female; would obscure
   essential anatomy)
6. True
7. Three
8. D. Within 1 minute following injection
9. B. Midway between xiphoid process
      and iliac crest
10. RPO
11. 30°
12. Erect position
13. The prostate gland will indent the
    floor of the bladder.
14. Just medial to the ASIS
15. Place the patient in a 15°
    Trendelenburg position.
16. A. Primarily the ureters
17. Renal pelvis, major and minor
    calyces of the kidneys
18. C. 10° to 15° caudad
19. True
20. 30° RPO

Review Exercise F: Problem Solving for Technical and Positioning Errors

1. A second projection of the bladder
   should be taken, using a smaller IR
   placed crosswise to include this
   region. The larger IR should be centered 1 or 2 inches (2 to 5 cm)
   higher to include the upper
   abdomen.
2. Too long of a delay between the
   injection of contrast media and the

imaging of the nephrogram. The
nephrogram needs to be taken no
later than 60 seconds following injection.
3. Decrease the obliquity of the RPO to
   no more than 30°.
4. Place the pneumatic paddles just
   medial to the ASIS to allow for compression of the distal ureters against
   the pelvic brim.
5. Increase caudad angulation of the
   central ray to project the symphysis
   pubis below the bladder.
6. Decrease the span of time between
   projections to capture all phases of
   the urinary system. (Take images at
   1, 2, and 3 minutes rather than 1, 5,
   and 15 minutes.)
7. The technologist should not perform
   the compression phase of the study.
   Ureteric compression is contraindicated when an abdominal aortic
   aneurysm is suspected. (The technologist should consult with the
   radiologist or physician.)
8. The erect prevoid AP projection will
   best demonstrate an enlarged
   prostate gland.
9. Ultrasound or CT
10. CT is preferred, but a nuclear medi-
    cine procedure could also be per-
    formed.
11. The patient should be asked
    whether he is taking Glucophage. If
    the response is yes, then ask
    whether he has been off the drug
    for at least 48 hours. Document and
    inform the radiologist of the
    patient's condition and medication
    history prior to injection.
12. These are expected side effects, and
    the technologist should reassure the
    patient. No medical treatment is
    required.

17

SELF-TEST

My Score = _____ %

Directions: This self-test should be taken only after completing all of the readings, review exercises, and laboratory activities for a particular section. The purpose of this test is not only to provide a good learning exercise but also to serve as a good indicator of what your final evaluation exam will be. It is strongly suggested that if you do not get at least a 90% to 95% grade on this self-test, you review those areas in which you missed questions before going to your instructor for the final evaluation exam for this chapter. (There are 77 questions or blanks—each is worth 1.3 points.)

1. The kidneys are _____ structures.

   A. Retroperitoneal   B. Intraperitoneal   C. Infraperitoneal   D. Extraperitoneal

2. The ureters enter the _____ aspect of the bladder.

   A. Lateral   B. Anterolateral   C. Posterolateral   D. Superolateral

3. The kidneys lie on the _____ (**anterior** or **posterior**) surface of each psoas major muscle.

4. The kidneys lie at a _____ angle in relation to the coronal plane.

5. The three constricted points along the length of the ureters where a kidney stone is most likely to lodge are:

   A. _____   C. _____

   B. _____

6. An abnormal drop of more than _____ inches, or _____ cm, in the position of the kidneys when the patient is erect indicates a condition termed nephroptosis.

7. The buildup of nitrogenous waste in the blood creates a condition called _____ .

8. How much urine is normally produced by the kidneys in 24 hours?

   A. 2.5 liters   B. 180 liters   C. 0.5 liter   D. 1.5 liters

9. The renal veins connect directly to the:

   A. Abdominal aorta   C. Azygos vein

   B. Superior mesenteric vein   D. Inferior vena cava

10. The 8 to 18 conical masses found within the renal medulla are called the _____ .

11. The major calyces of the kidney unite to form the _____ .

12. The microscopic unit of the kidney (of which there are over a million in each kidney) is called the

    _____ .

13. True/False: The loop of Henle and collecting tubules are located primarily in the medulla of the kidney.

14. True/False: About 50% of the glomerular filtrate processed by the nephron is reabsorbed into the kidney's venous system.

15. The inner, posterior triangular aspect of the bladder that is attached to the floor of the pelvis is called the

    _____ .

17

16. Identify the structures labeled on this radiograph (Fig. 17-4):

    A. _____

    B. _____

    C. _____

    D. _____

    E. _____

    F. _____

17. The term describing the radiographic procedure demonstrated on the radiograph in Fig. 17-4 is

    _____.

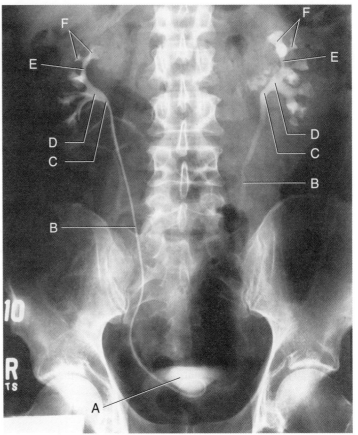

Fig. 17-4. Radiograph of the urinary system.

18. Under what circumstances should a pregnant patient have an IVU performed?

    _____

19. List the two classes of iodinated contrast media used for urinary studies. _____

20. Match the following characteristics to the correct type of iodinated contrast media:

    _____ A. Dissociates into two separate ions once injected   I. Ionic

    _____ B. Possesses low osmolality   N. Nonionic

    _____ C. Uses a salt as its cation

    _____ D. Parent compound is a carboxyl group

    _____ E. Less expensive of the two types

    _____ F. Produces a less severe contrast media reaction

    _____ G. Diatrizoate is a common anion

    _____ H. Does not contain a cation

    _____ I. Creates a hypertonic condition in blood plasma

    _____ J. Creates a near isotonic solution

21. The normal range of creatinine in an adult is:

    A. 2.0 to 3.4 mg/dl   C. 8 to 25 mg/100 ml

    B. 0.6 to 1.5 mg/dl   D. 0.1 to 1.25 mg/dl

22. How long must a patient be withheld from Glucophage before and following an iodinated contrast media procedure?

    A. 48 hours   C. 24 hours

    B. 2 hours   D. 72 hours

23. Which one of the following conditions is considered high risk for an iodinated contrast media procedure?

    A. Hematuria   C. Diabetes mellitus

    B. Pheochromocytoma   D. Hypertension

24. What is the best course of action for a patient experiencing a mild level contrast media reaction?

    A. Observe and reassure patient   C. Inform your supervisor

    B. Call for immediate medical attention   D. Inform the referring physician

25. A reaction based on fear or anxiety is classified as a(n):

    A. Vasomotor effect   C. Anaphylactic reaction

    B. Vasovagal reaction   D. Anxiety attack

26. A true allergic reaction to iodinated contrast agents is classified as a(n):

    A. Vasomotor effect   C. Anaphylactic reaction

    B. Vasovagal reaction   D. Acute renal failure

27. Tachycardia (> 100 beats/minute) is a symptom of a(n) _____ type of reaction.

    A. Vasomotor effect   C. Anaphylactic reaction

    B. Vasovagal reaction   D. Acute renal failure

28. Brachycardia (< 50 beats/minute) is a symptom of a(n) _____ type of reaction.

    A. Vasomotor effect   C. Anaphylactic reaction

    B. Vasovagal reaction   D. Acute renal failure

29. Which of the following drugs may be given to reduce the risk for acute renal failure?

    A. Prednisone   C. Benadryl

    B. Corticosteroid   D. Lasix

30. Glucophage is a drug given to patients with:

    A. Sensitivity to iodine   C. Acute renal failure

    B. Diabetes   D. Chronic renal failure

31. Which one of the following drugs can be given as part of the premedication protocol prior to an iodinated contrast media procedure?

    A. Prednisone   C. Cipro

    B. Zantac   D. Pentobarbital

17

32. Excretion of a diminished amount of urine in relation to the fluid intake is the general definition for:

    A. Polyuria   C. Oliguria

    B. Proteinuria   D. Nephroptosis

33. Constant or frequent involuntary passage of urine is termed:

    A. Micturition   C. Retention

    B. Urinary reflux D. Urinary incontinence

34. The absence of a functioning kidney is called:

    A. Renal agenesis C. Nephroptosis

    B. Renal failure   D. Oliguria

35. Complete cessation of urinary secretion by the kidneys is termed:

    A. Micturition C. Urinary incontinence

    B. Anuria   D. Chronic renal failure

36. True/False: Adult forms of polycystic disease are inherent.

37. Hypernephroma is another term for:

    A. Renal cell carcinoma C. Hydronephrosis

    B. Wilms' tumor   D. Renal hypertension

38. Extravasation is classified as a:

    A. Side effect   C. Moderate level reaction

    B. Mild level reaction D. Severe level reaction

39. Profound shock is classified as a:

    A. Side effect   C. Moderate level reaction

    B. Mild level reaction D. Severe level reaction

40. Hot flashes are classified as a:

    A. Side effect   C. Moderate level reaction

    B. Mild level reaction D. Severe level reaction

41. Which one of the following veins is **not** normally selected for venipuncture during an IVU?

    A. Basilic   C. Axillary

    B. Cephalic   D. Radial

42. At what angle is the needle advanced into the vein during venipuncture? _____

43. The complete cessation of urinary secretion is called _____ .

44. A technique of using acoustic waves to shatter large kidney stones is called _____ .

45. The most common cause of urinary tract infection is:

    A. Renal calculi C. Urinary incontinence

    B. Uremia   D. Vesicourethral reflux

46. Which one of the following conditions may produce hydronephrosis?

    A. Renal obstruction   C. Renal hypertension

    B. Glomerulonephritis   D. BPH

47. Which one of the following pathologic indications is an example of a congenital anomaly of the urinary system?

    A. Ectopic kidney   C. Urinary tract infection

    B. Pyelonephritis   D. BPH

48. True/False: The patient should void before the IVU to prevent dilution of the contrast media in the bladder.

49. True/False: The patient should complete a bowel cleansing procedure before the IVU.

50. Which one of the following conditions would contraindicate the use of ureteric compression?

    A. Hematuria   C. Urinary tract infection

    B. Ureteric calculi   D. Multiple myeloma

51. Typically, at what timing sequence during an IVU are the oblique projections taken? _____

52. Which projection(s) best demonstrate(s) the renal parenchyma? When should it (they) be taken?

    _____

53. Which procedure may require a Brodney clamp? _____

54. Which specific body position will place the right kidney parallel to the IR? _____

55. True/False: The gonadal dose for the AP postvoid projection is higher for male patients than for female patients.

56. True/False: The retrograde ureterogram will demonstrate the ureters, renal pelvis, and major and minor calyces.

57. **Situation:** An AP projection taken during a retrograde cystogram reveals that the symphysis pubis is superimposed over the floor of the bladder. What can be done during the repeat exposure to correct this problem?

    _____

58. **Situation:** Prior to the beginning of an IVU, the radiologist requests a nephrogram be taken as part of the study. At what point of the study should this projection be taken?

    _____

59. **Situation:** A patient comes to the radiology department for an IVU following abdominal surgery the day before. The IVU protocol requires that ureteric compression be used. What else can be done to achieve the same goal without using compression?

    _____

60. **Situation:** A radiograph of a RPO position taken during an IVU reveals that the left kidney is foreshortened and superimposed over the spine. What is the positioning error that led to this radiographic outcome?

    _____

17

CHAPTER 18

Mammography

After you have successfully completed the activities in this chapter, you will be able to:

_____ 1. List statistics for breast cancer in the United States and worldwide.

_____ 2. Describe the recommendations from the American Cancer Society and American College of Radiology (ACR) in regard to mammography.

_____ 3. Describe the impact of the Mammography Quality Standards Act (MQSA) on mammography facilities and mammographers.

_____ 4. On drawings and radiographs, identify specific anatomy of the female breast.

_____ 5. Identify specific regions of the breast using the quadrant and the clock systems.

_____ 6. List the three general categories of breast tissue according to their tissue composition, age of the patient, and radiographic density.

_____ 7. Identify the three classifications of the breast.

_____ 8. Describe the general patient preparation concerns prior to a mammogram.

_____ 9. Identify key questions that should be asked as part of the clinical history taking prior to a mammogram.

_____ 10. List the technical considerations and equipment essential for quality images of the breast.

_____ 11. Identify the diagnostic benefits of breast compression and the average pounds of force used when applying compression.

_____ 12. Identify the principal way patient dose can be decreased or controlled during mammography.

_____ 13. Compare and contrast the advantages and disadvantages of film-screen and digital mammography.

_____ 14. List the benefits of using computed-aided detection (CAD) in mammographic interpretation.

_____ 15. Identify alternative imaging modalities available to study the breast, including advantages and disadvantages of each system.

_____ 16. Describe the basic and special projections most commonly performed in mammography; include patient positioning, CR placement, and structures best seen.

_____ 17. Describe the Eklund technique for imaging breasts with implants.

_____ 18. List the average skin dose and mean glandular dose (MGD) range for each projection of the breast as described in the textbook.

_____ 19. Define specific types of breast pathology.

_____ 20. List the American College of Radiology nomenclature of terms and abbreviations for mammographic positioning.

_____ 21. Given mammographic images, identify specific positioning and exposure factor errors.

Positioning and IR Critique

_____ 1. Using a peer in a simulated setting, position for basic and special mammographic projections.

_____ 2. Using appropriate radiographic phantoms, produce satisfactory radiographs of specific positions (if equipment is available).

_____ 3. Critique and evaluate mammographic images based on the four divisions of radiographic criteria: (1) structures shown, (2) position, (3) collimation and CR, and (4) exposure criteria.

_____ 4. Distinguish between acceptable and unacceptable mammographic images based on exposure factors, motion, collimation, positioning, or other errors.

Learning Exercises

The following review exercises should be completed only after careful study of the associated pages in the textbook as indicated by each exercise. Answers to each review exercise are given at the end of the review exercises.

Part I: Breast Cancer, Anatomy of the Breast, and Mammography Quality Standards

REVIEW EXERCISE A: Breast Cancer, Anatomy of the Breast, and Mammography Quality Standards Act (see textbook pp. 580-583)

1. Radiographic examination of the mammary gland or breast is called _____ .

2. In 1992 the American Cancer Society recommended that women over the age of _____

   should have a screening mammogram performed.

   A. 35   C. 45

   B. 40   D. 50

3. The Mammography Quality Standards Act (MQSA), which went into effect on October 1, _____ , was passed to ensure high-quality mammography service requiring certification by the secretary of the Department of Health and Human Services (DHHS).

   A. 1992   C. 1994

   B. 1993   D. 1995

4. There are over _____ documented cases of breast cancer worldwide.

5. Men have _____ % chance of developing breast cancer as compared with women.

6. Once a breast cancer tumor has reached a size of _____ cm, it has often metastasized.

7. As stated in the textbook, breast cancer accounts for _____ of all new cancers detected in women.

   A. 12%   C. 32%

   B. 15%   D. 50%

8 In Canada, mammography guidelines are set by the _____ .

9. Which of the following mammography facilities are exempt from MQSA standards?

   A. Medicare facilities   C. Not-for-profit facilities

   B. VA facilities   D. No facilities are exempt

10. The junction of the inferior part of the breast with the anterior chest wall is called the

    _____ .

11. The pigmented area surrounding the nipple is the _____ .

12. Breast tissue extending into the axilla is called the tail of the breast, or the _____ .

13. In the average female breast, the _____ (**craniocaudad** or **mediolateral**) diameter is
    usually greater.

14. Five o'clock on the right breast would be in what quadrant? _____

15. Based on the clock system method, a suspicious mass at 2 o'clock on the right breast would be a _____ o'clock
    if it were in a similar position on the left breast.

16. What is the large muscle commonly seen on a mammogram that is located between the bony thorax and the

    mammary gland? _____

17. Two fibrous sheets of tissue join together just posterior to the breast to form the _____
    space.

18. What is the function of the mammary gland? _____

19. List the three tissue types found in the female breast:

    A. _____   B. _____   C. _____

20. Various small blood vessels, fibrous connective tissues, ducts, and other small structures seen on finished

    mammograms are collectively called _____ .

21. Bands of connective tissue passing through the breast tissue are known as _____ .

22. Classify the following types of breasts into one of the three general categories: fibro-glandular (FG), fibro-fatty
    (FF), or fatty (F).

    _____ 1. 20 years, no children   _____ 5. 50 years, two children

    _____ 2. 35 years, no children   _____ 6. Male

    _____ 3. 35 years, three children   _____ 7. 35 years, lactating

    _____ 4. 25 years, pregnant   _____ 8. 10 years

23. Which is the least dense of the following tissues: fibrous, glandular, or adipose? _____

18

24. Identify the labeled parts on this sagittal section drawing (Fig. 18-1):

A. _____

B. _____

C. _____

D. _____

E. _____

F. _____

G. _____

H. _____

I. _____

J. _____

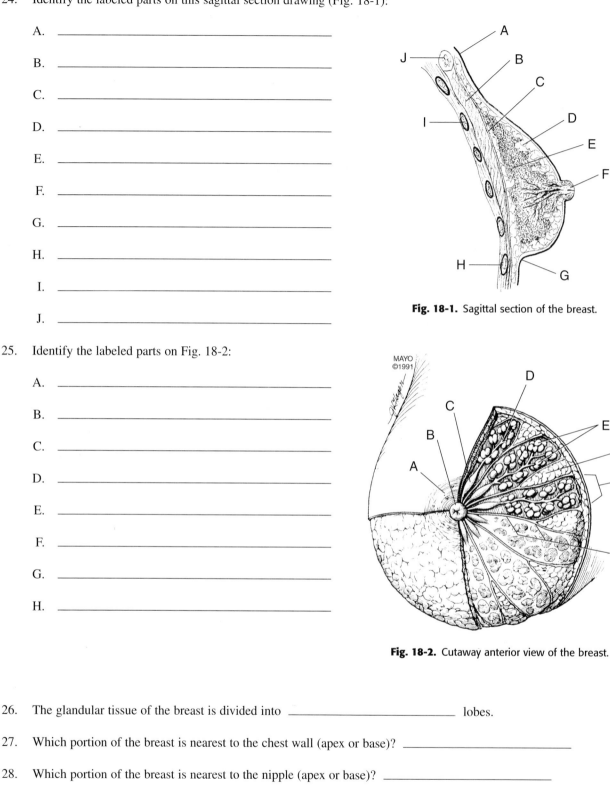

Fig. 18-1. Sagittal section of the breast.

25. Identify the labeled parts on Fig. 18-2:

A. _____

B. _____

C. _____

D. _____

E. _____

F. _____

G. _____

H. _____

Fig. 18-2. Cutaway anterior view of the breast.

26. The glandular tissue of the breast is divided into _____ lobes.

27. Which portion of the breast is nearest to the chest wall (apex or base)? _____

28. Which portion of the breast is nearest to the nipple (apex or base)? _____

29. The central ray is usually directed through the _____ of the breast.

30. What is the typical skin dose for a mammographic projection?

    A.   100 to 200 mrad   C.   800 to 1000 mrad

    B.   400 to 600 mrad   D.   1200 to 1500 mrad

31. To minimize patient dose, the ACR recommends a repeat rate of less than:

    A. 2%   C. 10%

    B. 5%   D. 15%

32. True/False: *MGD*, as used in patient dose measurements in mammography, refers to mean gonadal dose.

Part II: Patient Preparation, Technical Considerations, Alternative Modalities, and Radiographic Positioning

REVIEW EXERCISE B: Patient Preparation, Technical Considerations, Alternative Modalities, and Radiographic Positioning (see textbook pp. 584-595)

1. Other than jewelry and clothing, what substances must be removed from the patient's body prior to mammography to prevent artifacts?

    _____

2. What type of drinks should not be ingested by the patient prior to a mammogram?

    _____

3. What effect do the substances described in question 2 have on breast tissues?

    _____

4. List the six questions that should be included in the patient history taking prior to a mammogram:

    A. _____

    B. _____

    C. _____

    D. _____

    E. _____

    F. _____

5. True/False: Skin tattoos on the breast may produce an artifact on the image.

6. The ideal kilovoltage for mammography is between _____ and _____ kV.

7. Name the target material commonly used in mammography x-ray tubes: _____

8. The focal spot size on a dedicated mammography unit should be _____ mm or less.

9. Typically, compression applied to the breast is _____ to _____ pounds of pressure.

10. List the six benefits of applying breast compression during mammography:

    A. _____

    B. _____

    C. _____

D. _____

E. _____

F. _____

11. How does breast compression improve image quality or resolution?

A. _____

B. _____

12. The average required mAs range in mammography when using 25 to 28 kV is:

A. 10 to 15   C. 40 to 60

B. 20 to 30   D. 75 to 85

13. What is the three-part hallmark of good film-screen mammography (i.e., what are the three image qualities that need to be present on a diagnostic film-screen mammogram)?

A. _____   B. _____   C. _____

14. True/False: Grids and AEC are used for most mammograms.

15. True/False: Automatic exposure control should not be used with breast implants.

16. Magnification is performed during mammography primarily to:

A. Increase signal-to-noise ratio   C. Reduce dose per projection

B. Magnify specific regions of interest   D. Demonstrate the deep chest wall

17. What is the average mean glandular dose for projections of the breast?

A. 130 to 150 mrad   C. 500 to 700 mrad

B. 200 to 400 mrad   D. 900 to 1000 mrad

18. List the three advantages of computed radiographic mammography over conventional film-screen mammography:

A. _____

B. _____

C. _____

19. What is the name of the device that captures the image with direct digital mammography?

_____

20. True/False: Digital mammography can now match the overall spatial resolution produced with film-screen systems.

21. True/False: Computer-aided detection provides a "second opinion" on the interpretation of mammographic images.

22. What type of lesion is best diagnosed with sonography of the breast?

_____

23. Which imaging modality is most effective in diagnosing problems related to breast implants?

_____

24. List the two advantages of digital mammography over conventional film-screen systems:

A. _____

B. _____

25. A nuclear medicine procedure called **mammoscintigraphy** utilizes which radionuclide?

A. Cardiolyte   C. Thallium

B. Iodine 131   D. Sestamibi

26. A second type of nuclear medicine procedure called **sentinel node studies** is performed to:

A. Determine whether a malignant lesion is present in the breast

B. Detect malignant involvement of a lymph node surrounding the breast

C. Distinguish between a benign and a malignant tumor of the breast

D. Diagnose a lymphoma

27. What type of radionuclide is often used with sentinal node studies?

A. Sulfur colloid   C. Sestamibi

B. Technetium   D. FDG

28. PET studies of the breast can detect early cancerous cells by measuring the rate of:

A. Oxygen metabolism   C. Sugar metabolism

B. Phosphorus metabolism   D. Osmosis through the cell membrane

29. List the two major disadvantages of using PET as a breast screening tool:

A. _____

B. _____

30. True/False: MRI of the breast provides better diagnostic sensitivity and specificity as compared with ultrasound and conventional mammography.

31. True/False: MRI is less effective than conventional mammography in detecting lesions in the breast containing implants.

32. List the two primary disadvantages in using MRI to study the breast:

A. _____

B. _____

33. The most common form of benign tumor of the breast is:

A. Fibroadenoma   C. Fibrocystic lesion

B. Adenocarcinoma   D. Adenosarcoma

34. The most common form of breast cancer is:

A. Fibroadenoma   C. Infiltrating ductal carcinoma

B. Intraductal papilloma   D. Lobular carcinoma

35. Which of the following breast lesions has well-defined margins?

A. Gynecomastia   C. Fibroadenoma

B. Lobular carcinoma   D. Infiltrating ductal carcinoma

18

36. True/False: Gynecomastia primarily involves the male breast.

37. What are the two basic projections performed for screening mammograms?

    A. _____   B. _____

38. What surface landmark determines the correct height for placement of the image receptor for the craniocaudad

    projection? _____

39. Anatomic side markers and patient identification information need to be placed near the _____
    side of the breast.

40. In the craniocaudad projection, what structure must be in profile? _____

41. In the craniocaudad projection, the head should be turned _____ (**toward** or **away
    from**) the side being radiographed.

42. Which basic projection taken during a screening mammogram will demonstrate more of the pectoral muscle?

    _____

43. How much CR/IR angulation is used for an average-size breast for the mediolateral oblique projection?

    _____

44. The patient with a small, thin breast requires _____ (**more** or **less**) CR angulation with
    the mediolateral oblique projection as compared with the average-size breast.

45. For the mediolateral oblique projection, the arm of the side being examined should be placed:

    A. On the hip   C. Resting on top of the head

    B. Forward, toward the front of the body   D. Behind the back, palm out

46. Which special projection is usually requested when a lesion is seen on the mediolateral oblique but not on the

    craniocaudad projection? _____

47. In both the craniocaudad and the mediolateral projections, the central ray is generally directed to the

    _____ of the breast.

48. What is the most commonly requested special projection of the breast? _____

49. Which projection will most effectively show the axillary aspect of the breast? _____

50. How much is the CR/IR angled from vertical for the mediolateral, true lateral projection? _____

51. True/False: Mark each of the following statements either **T** for true or **F** for false.

_____ A. It is important for all skin folds to be smoothed out and all wrinkles and pockets of air removed on each projection for the breast.

_____ B. Since the base of the breast is well shown on the craniocaudad projection, this area does not need to be shown on the mediolateral oblique projection.

_____ C. The axillary aspect of the breast is usually well visualized on the craniocaudad projection.

_____ D. Mammography is usually done in the standing position.

_____ E. Because of a short exposure time, the patient does not need to be completely motionless during the exposure.

_____ F. Use of AEC would result in an underexposed image with breast implants.

_____ G. In the craniocaudad projection, the chest wall must be pushed firmly against the image receptor.

_____ H. Standard CC and MLO projections should be performed on patients who have breast implants.

_____ I. Firm compression should not be used on patients with breast implants.

_____ J. The patient skin dose for a true mediolateral projection is approximately 30% less than for the mediolateral oblique projection.

52. Which technique (method) is commonly used for the breast with an implant? _____

53. During the procedure identified in question 52, what must be done to allow the anterior aspect of the breast to be compressed and properly visualized?

_____

54. If a lesion is too deep toward the chest wall and cannot be visualized with a laterally exaggerated craniocaudal

projection, a(n) _____ projection should be performed.

A. Mediolateral oblique   C. Mediolateral

B. Craniocaudal   D. Axillary tail

55. Identify the correct positioning term or description for each of the following ACR abbreviations:

A. MLO _____   F. LM _____

B. SIO _____   G. XCCL _____

C. AT _____   H. LMO _____

D. CC _____   I. ID _____

E. RL _____

18

REVIEW EXERCISE C: Critique Radiographs of the Breast (see textbook p. 596)

These questions relate to the radiographs found at the end of Chapter 18 of the textbook. Evaluate these radiographs for the radiographic criteria categories (*1* through *5*) that follow. Describe the corrections needed to improve the overall image. The major, or "repeatable" errors, are specific errors that indicate the need for a repeat exposure, regardless of the nature of the other errors.

A. **CC projection (Fig. C18-40)**
   Description of possible error:

   1. Structures shown: _____

   2. Part positioning: _____

   3. Collimation and central ray: _____

   4. Exposure criteria: _____

   5. Markers: _____

   Repeatable error(s): _____

B. **MLO projection (Fig. C18-41)**
   Description of possible error:

   1. Structures shown: _____

   2. Part positioning: _____

   3. Collimation and central ray: _____

   4. Exposure criteria: _____

   5. Markers: _____

   Repeatable error(s): _____

C. **CC projection (Fig. C18-42)**
   Description of possible error:

   1. Structures shown: _____

   2. Part positioning: _____

   3. Collimation and central ray: _____

   4. Exposure criteria: _____

   5. Markers: _____

   Repeatable error(s): _____

D. **MLO projection (Fig. C18-43)**
   Description of possible error:

   1. Structures shown: _____

   2. Part positioning: _____

3. Collimation and central ray: _____

4. Exposure criteria: _____

5. Markers: _____

Repeatable error(s): _____

E. **CC projection (Fig. C18-44)**
    Description of possible error:

    1. Structures shown: _____

    2. Part positioning: _____

    3. Collimation and central ray: _____

    4. Exposure criteria: _____

    5. Markers: _____

    Repeatable error(s): _____

F. **CC projection (Fig. C18-45)**
    Description of possible error:

    1. Structures shown: _____

    2. Part positioning: _____

    3. Collimation and central ray: _____

    4. Exposure criteria: _____

    5. Markers: _____

    Repeatable error(s): _____

Part III: Laboratory Exercises

Exercise A below needs to be carried out in the radiology department where the mammography machine is located. Part B can be carried out in a classroom or any room where illuminators are available.

LABORATORY EXERCISE A: Positioning

For this section you need another person to act as your "patient." Male and female students should be separated for this exercise, and students can be fully clothed for the simulated positioning. A clinical instructor must be present. Include each of the following during this exercise (check off when completed):

_____ Manipulate the x-ray machine into all the positions and become familiar with the locks and devices.

_____ Place or exchange the cone on the x-ray machine.

_____ Place an IR into the cassette holder.

_____ Place a fist on the image receptor tray and compress it by using the compression device. (This should be performed so that the student can sense the pressure of the device.)

_____ Place another student in position and *simulate* the CC, MLO, XCCL, and ML positions.

_____ **Optional:** If the department or school has a breast phantom, perform the basic and special mammogram positions.

LABORATORY EXERCISE B: Image Critique and Evaluation

Your instructor will provide various breast radiographs for these exercises. Some will be optimal-quality radiographs that meet all or most of the evaluation criteria described for each projection in the textbook. Others will be of less than optimal quality, and others will be unacceptable, requiring a repeat exam. Evaluate each radiograph as specified below.

RADIOGRAPHS

1	2	3	4	5	6

_____ _____ _____ _____ _____ _____ a. Correct alignment and centering of part

_____ _____ _____ _____ _____ _____ b. Pectoral muscle included

_____ _____ _____ _____ _____ _____ c. Tissue thickness distributed evenly

_____ _____ _____ _____ _____ _____ d. Optimal compression noted

_____ _____ _____ _____ _____ _____ e. Dense areas adequately penetrated

_____ _____ _____ _____ _____ _____ f. High tissue contrast and optimal resolution noted

_____ _____ _____ _____ _____ _____ g. Absence of artifacts

_____ _____ _____ _____ _____ _____ h. Marker in proper position; accurate patient identification, including date

_____ _____ _____ _____ _____ _____ i. Based on acceptable variances to criteria factors, determine which of these radiographs are acceptable and which are unacceptable and should have been repeated. (Place a check mark if the radiograph needs to be repeated.)

Answers to Review Exercises

Review Exercise A: Breast Cancer, Anatomy of the Breast, and Mammography Quality Standards Act

1. Mammography
2. B. 40
3. C. 1994
4. 1 million
5. Between 1% and 2%
6. 2 cm
7. C. 32%
8. Canadian Association of Radiologists
9. B. VA facilities
10. Inframammary crease
11. Areola
12. Axillary prolongation
13. Mediolateral
14. Lower inner quadrant (LIQ)
15. 10 o'clock
16. Pectoralis major muscle
17. Retromammary
18. Lactation or secretion of milk
19. A. Glandular
    B. Fibrous or connective
    C. Adipose (fatty)
20. Trabeculae
21. Cooper's ligaments
22. 1. FG
    2. FG
    3. FF
    4. FG
    5. F
    6. F
    7. FG
    8. F
23. Adipose
24. A. Skin
    B. Pectoralis major muscle
    C. Retromammary space
    D. Adipose (fatty) tissue
    E. Glandular tissue
    F. Nipple
    G. Inframammary crease
    H. Sixth rib (lower breast margin— varies among individuals)
    I. Second rib (upper breast margin)
    J. Clavicle
25. A. Areola
    B. Nipple
    C. Ampulla
    D. Ducts
    E. Alveoli
    F. Mammary fat
    G. Lobe
    H. Cooper's ligament
26. 15 to 20
27. Base
28. Apex
29. Base
30. C. 800 to 1000 mrad
31. B. 5%
32. False (mean glandular dose)

Review Exercise B: Patient Preparation, Technical Considerations, Alternative Modalities, and Radiographic Positioning

1. Talcum powder and antiperspirant deodorant
2. Caffeinated drinks and those containing xanthine derivatives
3. They increase fluid retention in the breast, which limits visibility of breast tissue and increases discomfort during breast compression.
4. A. Possibility of pregnancy?
    B. Is there a family history of cancer including breast cancer?
    C. Medications currently taking?
    D. Previous surgery?
    E. Had previous mammogram?
    F. Any changes in breast, including lumps, pain, or discharge?
5. True
6. 25 to 28 kV
7. Molybdenum
8. 0.1 to 0.3 mm
9. 25 to 45
10. A. Decreases the thickness of the breast
    B. Brings the breast structures as close to the IR as possible
    C. Decreases dose and scattered radiation
    D. Decreases motion and geometric unsharpness
    E. Increases radiographic contrast
    F. Separates breast structure
11. A. Reduces scatter radiation
    B. Reduces magnification of breast structures
12. D. 75 to 85
13. A. Fine detail
    B. Edge sharpness
    C. Soft-tissue visibility
14. True
15. True
16. B. Magnify specific regions of interest
17. A. 130 to 150 mrad
18. A. Lower operating costs
    B. Can send images to remote locations via teleradiology
    C. Less physical storage space required (images can be archived and stored electronically in a PACS)
19. Flat detector
20. False
21. True
22. Distinguishing a cyst from a solid mass
23. Magnetic resonance imaging (MRI)
24. A. Mammographic images can be digitally enhanced, modified, or enlarged without additional exposure.
    B. Digital mammographic images can be sent to remote locations by telephone, satellite, or the Internet.
25. D. Sestamibi
26. B. Detect malignant involvement of a lymph node surrounding the breast
27. A. Sulfur colloid
28. C. Sugar metabolism
29. A. Cost
    B. Radiation exposure to the patient
30. True
31. False
32. A. High false, positive rate
    B. High cost
33. A. Fibroadenoma
34. C. Infiltrating ductal carcinoma
35. C. Fibroadenoma
36. True
37. A. Craniocaudal (CC)
    B. Mediolateral oblique (MLO)
38. Inframammary crease
39. Axillary
40. Nipple
41. Away from
42. Mediolateral oblique (MLO)
43. 45 degrees from vertical
44. More
45. B. Forward, toward the front of the body
46. Exaggerated craniocaudal (lateral), or XCCL
47. Base
48. Exaggerated craniocaudal (lateral), or XCCL
49. Exaggerated craniocaudal (lateral), or XCCL
50. 90 degrees
51. A. True
    B. False
    C. False
    D. True
    E. False
    F. False (overexposed)
    G. True
    H. True
    I. True
    J. False (same amount of dose)

18

52. Ecklund technique
53. The breast implant needs to be "pinched" or pushed posterior carefully toward the chest wall out of the exposure field.
54. D. Axillary tail
55. A. Mediolateral oblique
    B. Superolateral-inferomedial oblique
    C. Axillary tail
    D. Craniocaudal
    E. Rolled lateral
    F. Lateromedial
    G. Exaggerated craniocaudal (lateral)
    H. Lateromedial oblique
    I. Implant displaced

Review Exercise C: Critique Radiographs of the Breast

A. CC projection (Fig. C18-40)
   1. *Folds of fatty tissue superimpose breast tissue.
   2. Breast is not pulled away from chest wall; folds of tissue are not pulled back.
   3. Collimation is not applicable for mammography. CR centering is acceptable.
   4. Exposure factors are acceptable.
   5. Anatomic side marker is visible.
   Repeatable error(s): 1

B. MLO projection (Fig. C18-41)
   1. *Pertinent muscle is not seen to nipple level, and outer tissue is not compressed.
   2. Lower part of breast not pulled away from chest wall onto IR sufficiently.
   3. Collimation not applicable for mammography. CR centering is acceptable.
   4. Exposure factors are acceptable.
   5. Anatomic side marker is visible.
   Repeatable error(s): 1

C. CC projection (Fig. C18-42)
   1. *Part of posterior breast is cut off.
   2. *Medial posterior breast is not included, and shoulder is superimposed over the lateral posterior tissue.
   3. Collimation is not applicable for mammography. CR centering is acceptable.
   4. Exposure factors are acceptable.
   5. Anatomic side marker is visible.
   Repeatable error(s): 1 and 2

D. MLO projection (Fig. C18-43)
   1. *Posterior medial breast is cut off; no pectoral muscle is visible. (White specks are calcifications; they are not dust artifacts.)
   2. *Breast is not pulled out away from chest wall.

3. Collimation is not applicable for mammography. CR centering is acceptable.
   4. Exposure factors are acceptable.
   5. Anatomic side marker is visible.
   Repeatable error(s): 1 and 2

E. CC projection (Fig. C18-44)
   1. *Motion is present, which obliterates all detail.
   2. Acceptable—dark half-circle indicates posterior breast is included.
   3. Collimation is not applicable for mammography. CR centering is acceptable.
   4. Exposure factors are acceptable.
   5. Anatomic side marker is visible.
   Repeatable error(s): 1

F. CC projection (Fig. C18-45)
   1. *Hair artifacts are evident on posterior breast tissue, obscuring breast tissue detail.
   2. Acceptable.
   3. Collimation is not applicable for mammography. CR is slightly off-centered toward medial side.
   4. Exposure factors are acceptable.
   5. Anatomic side marker is visible.
   Repeatable error(s): 1

SELF-TEST

Directions: This self-test should be taken only after completing all of the readings, review exercises, and laboratory activities for a particular section. The purpose of this test is not only to provide a good learning exercise but also to serve as a good indicator of what your final evaluation exam will be. It is strongly suggested that if you do not get at least a 90% to 95% grade on this self-test, you review those areas in which you missed questions before going to your instructor for the final evaluation exam for this chapter. (There are 68 questions or blanks—each is worth 1.5 points.)

1.   What does the acronym *MQSA* represent, and what year did it go into effect? _____

     _____

2.   Which health facilities (if any) are exempt from the MQSA requirements? _____

3.   In 1992, the American Cancer Society recommended that all women over the age of _____ undergo annual screening mammography.

4.   Currently, 1 in _____ American women will develop breast cancer sometime during her life.

5.   The junction between the inferior aspect of the breast and chest wall is called the _____ .

6.   In which quadrant of the breast is the tail, or axillary prolongation, found? _____ .

7.   Using the clock system, one o'clock in the left breast would correspond to _____ in the right breast.

8.   Which large muscle is located directly posterior to the breast? _____

9.   What is the function of the mammary gland? _____

10. Name the bands of connective tissue passing through the breast tissue to provide support. _____

11. Which one of the three breast tissue types is the least dense radiographically? _____

12. What is the term used by radiologists for various small structures seen on the mammogram? _____

13. Which term describes the thickest portion of the breast near the chest wall? _____

14. Which one of the following tissue types would be found in the breasts of a 25-year-old pregnant female?

     A. Fibro-glandular   C. Fatty

     B. Fibro-fatty   D. Cystic

15. Which one of the following tissue types would be found in the breasts of a 35-year-old female who has borne two children?

     A. Fibro-glandular   C. Fatty

     B. Fibro-fatty   D. Cystic

16. The male breast would be classified as:

     A. Fibro-glandular   C. Fatty

     B. Fibro-fatty   D. Cystic

17. Which one of the following tissue types requires more compression during mammography as compared with the others?

    A. Fibro-glandular   C. Fatty

    B. Fibro-fatty   D. Cystic

18. Identify the anatomy labeled on Fig. 18-3:

    A. _____

    B. _____

    C. _____

    D. _____

    E. Which basic mammogram projection is demonstrated in

        Fig. 18-3? _____

    F. The right side marker on this mammogram is correctly

        placed on the _____ side
        of the breast.

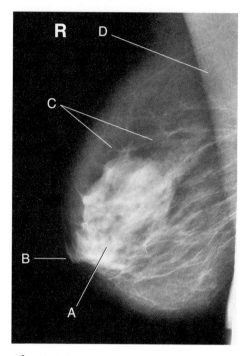

Fig. 18-3. Breast anatomy on a mammogram.

19. The target material used in most mammography x-ray tubes is _____ .

20. To utilize the maximum advantage of the anode-heel effect, the anode side of the x-ray tube should be over the

    _____ (**base** or **apex**) of the breast.

21. True/False: Automatic exposure control (AEC) can be used for most mammographic projections.

22. True/False: Compression of the breast will improve image quality by reducing scatter radiation.

23. True/False: A grid is generally not used for mammography.

24. What size focal spot should be used for magnification of small breast nodules or tissue samples? _____

25. What is the magnification factor for an exposure with a source object distance (SOD) of 20 inches and a source

    image receptor distance (SID) of 40 inches? _____

26. The average mean glandular dose received by the patient during a basic two-projection mammogram examination is
    in the range of:

    A. 50 to 150 mrad   C. 400 to 600 mrad

    B. 200 to 300 mrad   D. 800 to 1100 mrad

18

27. Which imaging modality is best suited to distinguish a cyst from a solid mass within the breast?

_____

28. Which imaging modality is best suited to diagnose an extracapsular rupture of a breast implant?

_____

29. True/False: Breast imaging using sonography has been performed since the mid-1970s.

30. True/False: The principal way to reduce patient dose during mammography is to use higher kV techniques.

31. True/False: One reason that mammoscintigraphy is not ordered more frequently is the high number of false positives reported with this procedure.

32. Which one of the following radionuclides is used for sentinel node studies?

A. Sulfur colloid   C. Technetium

B. Sestamibi   D. Iodine 131

33. Carcinoma of the breast is divided into two categories: _____ and _____ .

34. Which one of the following ACR abbreviations refers to the *exaggerated craniocaudal (lateral)* projection?

A. LECC   C. LCC

B. LXCC   D. XCCL

35. What is the ACR abbreviation for a *mediolateral oblique* projection? _____

36. List the two basic projections taken during a screening mammogram:

A. _____   B. _____

37. Which of the basic projections taken during a mammogram will best demonstrate the pectoral muscle?

_____

38. The typical kV range for mammography is _____ .

39. Which projection best demonstrates the axillary aspect of the breast? _____

40. What is the ACR abbreviation for the special projection, lateromedial oblique, used with a pacemaker?

_____

41. The use of AEC when performing a projection with a breast implant in place can lead to

_____ (**overexposure** or **underexposure**) of the breast.

42. A. The technique of "pinching" the breast to push an implant posteriorly to the chest wall is known as the

_____ technique.

B. What is the correct ACR term and abbreviation for this technique? _____

18

43. What other special projection can be taken if a lesion is too deep into the axillary tail aspect of the chest wall to be seen with an exaggerated craniocaudal projection? (Include the correct ACR term and abbreviation.)

_____

44. Identification markers should always be placed near the _____ .

45. How is the opposite breast prevented from superimposing the breast being examined on the MLO projection?

_____

46. With a large breast, which of the two basic projections is most likely to require two images to include all the breast

tissue? _____

47. Which projection is usually requested when a lesion is seen on the MLO (mediolateral oblique) but not on the CC

(craniocaudad) projection? _____

48. What landmark determines the correct height for placement of the image receptor for the CC (craniocaudad)

projection? _____

49. Which one of the following projections is recommended for demonstrating inflammation of the breast?

   A. Craniocaudal   C. Mediolateral (true lateral)

   B. Mediolateral oblique   D. Exaggerated craniocaudal (lateral)

50. **Situation:** A mammogram is performed for a patient with breast implants. The resultant images are overexposed. The following factors were used: 28 kV, AEC, grid, and gentle compression. Which one of the following modifications would produce more diagnostic images during the repeat study?

   A. Lower the kV   C. Use manual exposure factors

   B. Do not use a grid   D. Do not use breast compression

51. What device or system is part of direct digital mammography?

   A. Imaging plate   C. Bucky tray

   B. Image intensifier   D. Flat panel receptor

52. True/False: The spatial resolution of digital mammography currently equals that of film-screen imaging.

53. CAD is an acronym for _____ .

54. It is reported that CAD can improve breast cancer detection rate by _____ %.

55. What type of radionuclide is used with mammoscintigraphy?

   A. Technetium-99m-sestamibi   C. Sulfur colloid

   B. Iodine 131   D. Gadolinium

56. PET scanning can detect early cancer cells by their increased _____ .

57.   True/False: Patient dose from a PET scan of the breast is comparable to that with an film-screen mammogram.

58.   Which of the following imaging modalities is most effective in studying the breast with implants?

A.   Ultrasound   C.   MRI

B.   PET   D.   IR-screen mammography

59.   One of the major disadvantages of using MRI as a breast screening tool is:

A.   Higher patient dose   C.   Patient discomfort

B.   High false-positive rate   D.   Length of the exam

60.   The most common form of breast cancer is:

A.   Fibroadenoma   C.   Lobular carcinoma

B.   Infiltrating sarcoma   D.   Infiltrating ductal carcinoma

CHAPTER 19

Trauma, Mobile, and Surgical Radiography

This chapter has been divided into the following five sections:

1. **Trauma and Fracture Terminology.** Technologists should know the more common fracture terms included in this chapter to better understand patient histories and to ensure that the most appropriate projections are taken to demonstrate these fracture sites.
2. **Positioning Principles and Grid Use.** Understanding certain positioning principles, including correct use of portable grids, is essential in trauma and mobile radiography as it is described in this section.
3. **Mobile X-Ray Equipment and Radiation Protection.** Understanding the various types of mobile x-ray and fluoroscopy equipment used in trauma radiography (including use in surgery) is essential for technologists. Knowing and following safe radiation protection practices for workers around mobile equipment is especially important because of the unshielded environments where mobile equipment is generally used (such as in the emergency room, in surgery, or in patients' rooms).
4. **Trauma and Mobile Positioning and Procedures.** This section describes specific positioning for each body part in which the patient cannot be moved from the supine position. Adaptation of CR angles and IR placement as required is demonstrated and described for each body part.
5. **Surgical Radiography.** This section describes the role and responsibilities of the radiologic technologist in performing imaging in the surgical suite. Included are the following: essential surgical terminology, surgical radiographic equipment, various orthopedic fixation devices, and common surgical procedures that require radiographic support.

CHAPTER OBJECTIVES

After you have successfully completed the activities of this chapter, you will be able to:

_____ 1. Define and apply terms for specific types of fractures and soft-tissue injuries.

_____ 2. List the projections taken for a postreduction study of the limbs, including open and closed reductions.

_____ 3. Explain the two positioning principles that must be observed during trauma radiography.

_____ 4. List the three grid use rules to prevent cutoff.

_____ 5. Describe the two primary types of mobile radiographic units and their operating principles.

_____ 6. Explain the features, operating principles, and uses of mobile fluoroscopy units.

_____ 7. List the three methods for maintaining a sterile field with C-arm equipment.

_____ 8. List the three cardinal rules of radiation protection as they apply to trauma and mobile radiography.

_____ 9. Describe the difference in exposure field levels with different orientations of the x-ray tube and intensifiers with the C-arm.

_____ 10. Explain why the AP projection orientation of the C-arm is not recommended.

_____ 11. List projections for trauma and mobile procedures of the chest, bony thorax, and abdomen.

_____ 12. List projections for trauma and mobile procedures for various parts of the upper and lower limbs.

_____ 13. List projections for trauma and mobile procedures of the cervical, thoracic, and lumbar spine.

_____ 14. List trauma and mobile procedures for the skull and facial bones.

_____ 15. List the essential attributes of an effective surgical technologist.

_____ 16. Describe the role of the various members of the surgical team.

_____ 17. Differentiate between sterile and nonsterile environments in the surgical suite.

_____ 18. Define *asepsis* and describe methods and procedures to protect the integrity of the sterile environment.

_____ 19. Describe surgical garb that must be worn by the technologist prior to entering the operating suite, presurgical area, and recovery.

_____ 20. Explain the preparation, cleaning, and safe use of radiographic equipment in surgery.

_____ 21. Describe common radiographic procedures performed in surgery, including required equipment, the role of the technologist, and surgical equipment and devices used during the procedure.

_____ 22. Match common surgical terms, orthopedic devices, and procedures to their correct definitions.

Learning Exercises

The following review exercises should be completed only after careful study of the associated pages in the textbook as indicated by each exercise. Answers to each review exercise are given at the end of the review exercises.

REVIEW EXERCISE A: Radiographic Trauma and Fracture Terminology (see textbook pp. 598-599)

1. True/False: Mobile CT units are available for use in emergency and surgical situations.

2. True/False: Nuclear medicine is effective in diagnosing certain emergency conditions such as pulmonary emboli.

3. True/False: For trauma patients who cannot be moved for conventional diagnostic imaging, other modalities, such as ultrasound or nuclear medicine, may be used rather than trying to move the patient into specific positions.

4. List the two terms for describing displacement of a bone from a joint:

   A. _____   B. _____

5. List the four regions of the body most commonly dislocated during trauma:

   A. _____   C. _____

   B. _____   D. _____

6. What is the correct term for a partial dislocation? _____

7. A forced wrenching or twisting of a joint that results in a tearing of supporting ligaments is a _____ .

8. An injury in which there is no fracture or breaking of the skin is called a _____ .

9. What is the correct term that describes the relationship of the long axes of fracture fragments? _____

10. Which term describes a type of fracture in which the fracture fragment ends are overlapped and not in contact?

   _____

11. A. Which term describes the angulation of a distal fracture fragment toward the midline? _____

   B. Would this fracture angulation be described as a **medial** or **lateral** apex? _____

12. What is the primary difference between a simple and compound fracture?

   _____

19

13. List two types of incomplete fractures:

    A. _____   B. _____

14. Which type of comminuted fracture produces several wedge-shaped separate fragments? _____

15. What is the name of the fracture in which one fragment is driven into the other? _____

16. List the secondary name for the following fractures:

    A. Hutchinson's fracture: _____

    B. Baseball fracture: _____

    C. Compound fracture: _____

    D. Depressed fracture: _____

    E. Simple fracture: _____

17. True/False: An avulsion fracture is the same as a chip fracture.

18. What type of reduction fracture does *not* require surgery? _____

19. Match each of the following types of fractures to its correct definition (use each choice only once):

    _____   1. Greenstick   A. Fracture of proximal half of ulna with dislocation of radial head

    _____   2. Comminuted   B. Fracture of the base of the first metacarpal

    _____   3. Monteggia's   C. Fracture of the pedicles of C2

    _____   4. Boxer's   D. Fracture of distal radius with anterior displacement

    _____   5. Smith's   E. Complete fracture of distal fibula, frequently with fracture of medial malleolus

    _____   6. Hutchinson's   F. Fracture of lateral malleolus, medial malleolus, and distal posterior tip of tibia

    _____   7. Bennett's   G. Incomplete fracture with broken cortex on one side of bone only

    _____   8. Avulsion   H. Fracture resulting in multiple (two or more) fragments

    _____   9. Depressed   I. Fracture of distal fifth metacarpal

    _____   10. Stellate   J. Intraarticular fracture of radial styloid process

    _____   11. Trimalleolar   K. Fracture of distal radius with posterior displacement

    _____   12. Compression   L. Indented fracture of the skull

    _____   13. Pott's   M. Fracture due to a severe stress to a tendon

    _____   14. Colles'   N. Fracture with fracture lines radiating from center point

    _____   15. Hangman's   O. Fracture producing a reduced height of the anterior vertebral body

19

20. A. Fig. 19-1 illustrates which specific "named fracture?"

    _____

    B. Which bone is most commonly fractured, and which displacement commonly occurs with this fracture?

    _____

    C. Describe the type of injury or fall that commonly results

    in this type of fracture. _____

    _____

21. A. Fig. 19-2 illustrates which specific "named" fracture?

    _____

    B. Which bone(s) is(are) commonly fractured with this

    type of fracture? _____

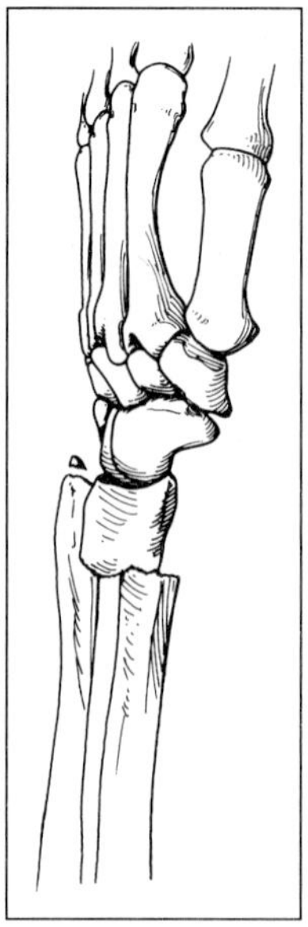

Fig. 19-1. 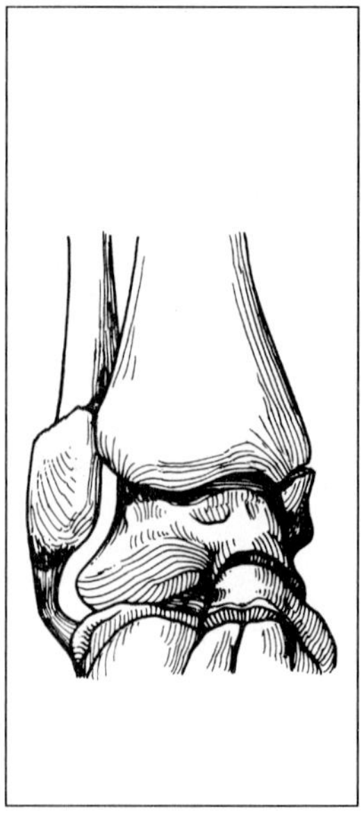 **Fig. 19-2.**

REVIEW EXERCISE B: Positioning Principles and Grids (see textbook pp. 603-605)

1. Which single term best describes the primary difference between trauma positions and standard positioning?

   _____

2. What should be done to achieve specific projections if the patient cannot move because of trauma?

   _____

3. What is the minimum number of projections generally required for any trauma study? _____

4. How many joints must be included for an initial study of a long bone? _____

5. True/False: A follow-up postreduction radiograph of the middle portion of long bones should be collimated closely to the fracture region.

6. Grids are required for any body part measuring greater than _____ cm.

7. List the three factors that must be met to avoid grid cutoff (three limitations or rules to prevent grid cutoff):

   A. _____ B. _____ C. _____

8. True/False: Lead grid lines usually run parallel to the centerline of the long axis of the grid.

9. True/False: To avoid grid cutoff, the angulation of the CR must be perpendicular to the length of the grid.

10. What does "grid focal range" mean? _____

11. What is the preferred grid ratio for a grid used for portable procedures? _____

12. What is considered to be a medium grid focal range? _____

13. A typical long focal range portable grid has a focal range of _____ .

14. What happens to the radiographic image if the SID exceeds a grid's focal range? _____ .

15. True/False: One particular surface of a focused grid must always be facing the x-ray tube to prevent grid cutoff.

16. A common grid ratio used for mobile work is:

      A.   4:1   B.   6:1 or 8:1   C.   10:1 or 12:1   D.   16:1

REVIEW EXERCISE C: Mobile X-Ray Equipment and Radiation Protection (see textbook pp. 606-609)

1. List the two primary types of mobile x-ray units:

      A. _____   B. _____

2. Which type of mobile unit is lighter in weight? _____

3. With battery-powered types, how long does recharging take if the batteries are fully discharged? _____

4. True/False: A fully charged battery-powered mobile unit has a driving range of up to 10 miles per hour on level ground.

5. What is the common term for a mobile fluoroscopy unit? _____

6. What are the two primary components of a mobile fluoroscopy unit (located on each end of the structure from which it gets its name)?

      A. _____   B. _____

7. Why shouldn't the mobile fluoroscopy unit be placed in the AP projection ("tube on top" position)?

      _____

8. A.   With the tube and intensifier in a horizontal position, at which side of the patient should the surgeon stand if

         he or she must remain near the patient—the x-ray tube side or the intensifier side? _____

      B.   Why? _____

9. Of the two monitors found on most mobile fluoroscopy units, which one is generally considered the "active"

      monitor—the right or the left? _____

10. True/False: Image orientation on the mobile fluoroscopy monitors must be determined by the operator *before* the patient is brought into the room.

11. True/False: All mobile digital fluoroscopy units have the ability to magnify the image on the monitor during fluoroscopy.

12. True/False: The intermittent mode used during mobile fluoroscopy procedures is helpful during procedures to produce brighter images, but it results in significantly increased patient exposure.

13. True/False: Standard cassettes with conventional single-exposure radiographs can be used with most mobile fluoroscopy units.

14. True/False: AEC exposure systems are not feasible with mobile fluoroscopy.

15. Name the feature that allows an image to be held on the monitor while also providing continuous fluoroscopy imaging.

_____

16. List the three methods for maintaining a sterile field with the mobile fluoroscopy unit.

A. _____   C. _____

B. _____

17. List the three terms describing the cardinal rules of radiation protection:

A. _____   B. _____   C. _____

18. Which cardinal rule is *most* effective in reducing occupational exposure? _____

19. Which one of the following measures is most effective (and practical) in limiting exposure with mobile fluoroscopy?

   A. Limit C-arm procedures to surgery cases only

   B. Prevent nonradiologists from using the C-arm

   C. Use intermittent or "foot-tapping" fluoroscopy

   D. Limit all fluoroscopy procedures to no more than 10 minutes

For Questions 20 to 24, review exposure field information on Figs. 19-3 and 19-4. Also see the same exposure field drawings and charts in Chapter 19 of the textbook.

20. **Situation:** The C-arm is in position for a PA projection. What exposure field range would the operator receive at waist level standing 3 feet from the patient?

   A. 20 to 25 mR/hr   C. 50 to 100 mR/hr

   B. 25 to 50 mR/hr   D. 100 to 300 mR/hr

21. Approximately how much exposure at waist level would the operator receive with 5 minutes of fluoroscopy exposure standing 3 feet from the patient? (HINT: First convert mR/hr to mR/min by dividing by 60; then multiply by minutes of fluoroscopy time.)

   A. 5 mR   C. 25 mR

   B. 60 mR   D. 2 mR

22. If a technologist receives 50 mR/hr standing 3 feet from the mobile fluoroscopy unit, what would be the exposure rate if he or she moved back to a distance of 4 feet?

   A. 10 mR/hr

   B. 25 mR/hr

   C. 100 mR/hr

   D. No significant difference

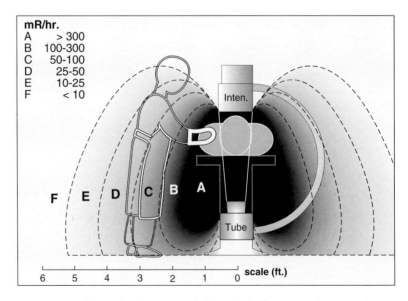

Fig. 19-3. Occupational exposure during mobile fluoroscopy, PA projection.

23. A technologist standing 1 foot from a mobile fluoroscopy unit is receiving approximately 400 mR/hr. What is the *total* exposure to the technologist if the procedure takes 10 minutes of fluoroscopy time to complete?

_____

24. **Situation:** An operator receives 25 mR/hr to the facial and neck region with the C-arm in position for a PA projection (intensifier on top). Approximately how much would the operator receive at the same distance if the C-arm were reversed to an AP projection position (tube on top)?

    A. 25 to 50 mR/hr

    B. 50 to 100 mR/hr

    C. 100 to 300 mR/hr

    D. 300 to 500 mR/hr

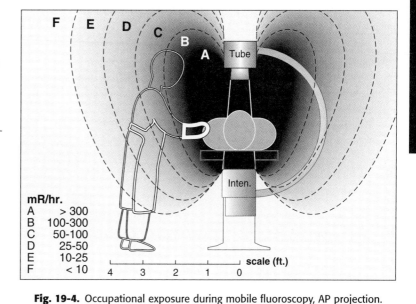

mR/hr.
A	> 300
B	100-300
C	50-100
D	25-50
E	10-25
F	< 10

Fig. 19-4. Occupational exposure during mobile fluoroscopy, AP projection.

25. A 30° C-arm tilt from the vertical perspective will increase exposure to the head and neck regions of the operator

    by a factor of _____ .

REVIEW EXERCISE D: Trauma and Mobile Positioning and Procedures (see textbook pp. 610-631)

1. How is the CR centered and aligned in relationship to the sternum for an AP portable projection of the chest?

   _____

2. True/False: Focused grids are recommended for mobile chest projections.

3. A.   A 35- × 43-cm (14- × 17-inch) IR should be placed _____ (**crosswise** or **lengthwise**) for an AP portable chest on an average or large patient.

   B.   Why? _____

4. What specific position should be performed to demonstrate a possible pneumothorax in the left lung for a patient

   who cannot stand or sit erect? _____

5. Which position can be used to replace the RAO of the sternum for the patient who cannot lie prone on the table but

   can be rotated into a semisupine position? _____

6. How must the grid be aligned to prevent grid cutoff when angling the CR mediolaterally for an oblique projection of the sternum when the patient cannot be rotated or moved at all from the supine position?

   _____

7. Other than the straight AP, what other projection of the ribs can be taken for the supine immobile patient who cannot be rotated into an oblique position? _____

8. Which one of the following positions or projections will best demonstrate free intra-abdominal air on the patient who cannot stand or sit erect?

   A. Left lateral decubitus   C. Right lateral decubitus

   B. AP KUB   D. Dorsal decubitus

9. Which one of the following projections of the abdomen will most effectively demonstrate a possible abdominal aortic aneurysm?

   A. Left lateral decubitus   C. Right lateral decubitus

   B. AP KUB   D. Dorsal decubitus

10. What is the disadvantage of performing a PA rather than an AP projection of the thumb?

    _____

11. Which projections are taken for a postreduction study of the wrist? _____

12. **Situation:** A study of a fractured wrist was taken with the following exposure factors: 60 kV, 10 mAs, detail screens. A fiberglass cast is placed on the wrist, and a postreduction study is ordered. Which one of the following techniques would be ideal for the postreduction study?

    A. 70 kV and 10 mAs   C. 65 kV and 10 mAs

    B. 80 kV and 10 mAs   D. 55 kV and 15 mAs

13. True/False: A PA horizontal beam projection of the elbow can be taken for a patient with multiple injuries.

14. True/False: For a trauma lateral projection of the elbow, the CR must be kept parallel to the interepicondylar plane.

15. **Situation:** A patient with a possible fracture of the proximal humerus enters the emergency room. Because of multiple injuries, the patient is unable to stand or sit erect. What positioning routine should be performed to diagnose the extent of the injury?

    _____

16. **Situation:** A patient with a possible dislocation of the proximal humerus enters the emergency room. Because of multiple injuries, the patient is unable to stand or sit erect. In addition to a basic AP projection, what second projection will demonstrate whether it is an anterior or posterior dislocation?

    _____

17. How much CR angulation should be used for an AP axial projection of the clavicle on a hypersthenic patient?

    A. 10°   B. 15°   C. 20°   D. 25°

18. A scapular "Y" projection taken AP for a trauma patient usually requires a _____ degree rotation of the body away from the image receptor.

    A. 20 to 30   B. 45   C. 50 to 60   D. 70

19. To ensure that the joints are opened up for an AP projection of the foot, how is the CR aligned?

    A. Perpendicular to the long axis of the tibia

    B. Perpendicular to the plantar surface

    C. 10° posteriorly from perpendicular to plantar surface

    D. 10° posteriorly from perpendicular to dorsal surface

20. **Situation:** An orthopedic surgeon orders a mortise projection of the ankle, but the patient has a severely fractured ankle and cannot rotate the ankle medially for the mortise projection. What can the technologist do to provide this projection without rotating the ankle?

_____

21. **Situation:** A patient with a possible dislocation of the patella enters the emergency room. What type of positioning routine should be performed on this patient that would safely demonstrate the patella?

_____

22. **Situation:** A patient with a possible fracture of the proximal tibia and fibula enters the emergency room. The basic AP and lateral projections are inconclusive. Because of severe pain, the patient is unable to rotate the leg from the AP position. What position or projection could be performed that would provide an unobstructed view of the fibular head and neck?

_____

23. Which one of the following positions would be performed on a trauma patient to provide a lateral view of the proximal femur?

    A. Danelius-Miller method   C. Waters method

    B. Fuchs method   D. Ottonello method

24. Which lateral projection can be taken of the proximal femur without having to abduct or flex the unaffected limb?

    _____

25. How is the CR aligned for the method identified in question 24?

_____

26. **Situation:** A patient with injuries suffered in a motor vehicle accident enters the emergency room. The ER physician orders a lateral C-spine projection to rule out a fracture or dislocation. Because of the thickness of the shoulders, C6-7 is not visualized. What additional projection can be taken safely to demonstrate this region of the spine?

_____

27. **Situation:** A patient with a possible C2 fracture enters the emergency room on a backboard. The AP projection does not demonstrate C2. In addition, the patient cannot open his mouth because of a mandible fracture. Which projection can be performed safely to demonstrate this region of the spine?

    A. Fuchs   C. Vertebral arch projection

    B. Judd   D. 35° to 40° cephalad axial projection

28. Which projection will best demonstrate (with only minimal distortion) the pedicles of the cervical spine on a severely injured patient?

_____

29. Identify the two CR angles for the double-angle Method Two for the oblique cervical spine:

    A. _____ ° medial   B. _____° cephalad

30. When using Method Two, double-angle technique, how is the cassette positioned for an oblique cervical spine to minimize distortion?

_____

31. **Situation:** A patient with a possible basilar skull fracture enters the emergency room. The ER physician wants a projection that best demonstrates a sphenoid effusion. The patient cannot stand or sit erect. Which one of the following projections would achieve this goal?

    A. AP skull

    B. Lateral recumbent skull

    C. Horizontal beam lateral skull

    D. Modified Waters projection

32. Which one of the following projections of the skull would project the petrous ridges in the lower one-third of the orbits on a supine trauma patient?

    A. AP skull, CR 0° to OML

    B. AP skull, CR 15° caudad to OML

    C. AP skull, CR 15° cephalad to OML

    D. AP skull, CR 30° caudad to OML

33. True/False: AP projections of the skull and facial bones will increase exposure to the thyroid gland as compared with PA projections.

34. True/False: The CR should not exceed a 30° caudad angle for the AP axial projection of the cranium to avoid excessive distortion of the cranial bones.

35. How is the CR angled and where is it centered for the AP acanthioparietal (reverse Waters) projection of the facial bones?

    _____

36. What type of CR angulation is required for the trauma version of an axiolateral projection of the mandible?

    _____

37. **Situation:** A patient with a Monteggia's fracture enters the emergency room. Which one of the following positioning routines should be performed on this patient?

    A. AP and lateral thumb

    B. PA and horizontal beam lateral wrist

    C. AP and horizontal beam lateral lower leg

    D. PA or AP and horizontal beam lateral forearm

38. **Situation:** A patient with a possible greenstick fracture enters the emergency room. What age group does this type of fracture usually affect?

    A. Pediatric

    B. Young adult

    C. Middle age

    D. Elderly

39. **Situation:** A patient with a possible Pott's fracture enters the emergency room. Which one of the following positioning routines should be performed on this patient?

    A. AP and horizontal beam lateral lower leg

    B. PA and horizontal beam lateral wrist

    C. AP and lateral thumb

    D. Three projections of the hand

40. **Situation:** A patient is struck directly on the patella with a heavy object, shattering it. The resultant fracture most likely would be described as a:

    A. Burst fracture

    B. Compression fracture

    C. Stellate fracture

    D. Smith's fracture

REVIEW EXERCISE E: Surgical Radiography (pp. 632-652)

1. List the four essential attributes of the successful surgical technologist:

    A. _____   C. _____

    B. _____   D. _____

2. Match the following roles to the correct member of the surgical team:

    _____ A. Individuals who assists the surgeon

    _____ B. Health-professional that prepares the OR by supplying it   1. Scrub
                with the appropriate supplies and instruments.
                                                                               2. Surgical assistant

    _____ C. Individual who has the responsibility of ensuring
                the safety of the patient and monitoring physiologic   3. Certified surgical
                functions and fluid levels of the patient during surgery   technologist

    _____ D. Individual who has primary responsibility for the   4. Surgeon
                surgical procedure and the well-being of the patient
                before, during, and immediately after surgery   5. Circulator

    _____ E. Individual who prepares the sterile field, scrubs and   6. Anesthesiologist
                gowns the members of the surgical team, and prepares
                and sterilizes the instruments before the surgical procedure

    _____ F. Individual who assists in the OR by responding to the needs
                of the scrubbed members within the sterile field before,
                during, and after the surgical procedure.

3. True/False: The technologist may violate the sterile environment in surgery if wearing sterile gloves, mask, and surgical scrubs.

4. True/False: The anesthesiologist works within the sterile environment.

5. True/False: The technologist has a moral and ethical responsibility to report any violations of the sterile field during surgery even if it was not noticed by another member of the surgical team.

6. True/False: The entire OR table is considered to be sterile.

7. List the three measures that can be taken to maintain the sterile field when operating a mobile fluoroscopy unit in a surgical suite:

    A. _____

    B. _____

    C. _____

8. Surgical _____ is the absence of infectious organisms.

9. Which parts of a sterile gown are considered sterile?

    A. From the top of the shoulders to the knee

    B. The sleeves and waist region

    C. The shoulders to the level of the sterile field, as well as the sleeve from the cuff to just above the elbow

    D. The entire surgical gown

10. _____ consists of the practice and procedures to minimize the level of infectious agents present in the surgical environment.

    A. Asepsis   C. Sterile practice

    B. OSHA standards   D. Surgical asepsis

11. True/False: Soft (canvas) shoes should be worn in surgery.

12. True/False: The pliable nose stripe on the surgical mask helps prevent fogging of eye glasses.

13. True/False: Protective eyewear is not required to be worn by the technologist during most surgical procedures.

14. True/False: Sterile gloves must be worn when handling a contaminated IR in surgery.

15. What type of equipment cleaner should **not** be used in surgery? _____

16. What is the primary disadvantage of using the "boost" feature during a mobile fluoroscopic procedure?

    _____

17. What is the primary advantage of using the "boost" feature during a mobile fluoroscopic procedure?

    _____

18. Which one of the following measures will best reduce dose to the patient and surgical team during a C-arm procedure?

    A. Reduce distance between anatomy and image intensifier

    B. Increase distance between anatomy and image intensifier

    C. Operate x-ray tube in vertical position above patient

    D. Operate x-ray tube in boost mode

19. What anatomy is examined during an operative (immediate) cholangiogram?

    _____

20. What is the common name for the special tray device that holds the IR and grid during an operative cholangiogram?

    _____

21. How must the IR and grid be aligned if the OR table is tilted during an operative cholangiogram?

    _____

22. On the average, how much contrast media is injected during an operative cholangiogram? _____

23. List the three advantages to laparoscopic cholecystectomy over traditional cholecystectomy:

    A. _____

    B. _____

    C. _____

24. A radiographic examination of the pelvicalyceal system only during surgery is termed:

    A. Retrograde ureterogram

    B. Antegrade pyelogram

    C. Nephrostomy

    D. Retrograde pyelogram

25. In what position is the patient placed during retrograde urography?

    A. Sims' position

    B. Modified lithotomy position

    C. Trendelenburg position

    D. Fowler's position

26. Which of the following orthopedic procedures is considered nonsurgical?

    A. Open reduction

    B. External fixation

    C. Closed reduction

    D. Internal fixation

27. Which of the following orthopedic devices is classified as an external fixator?

    A. Intramedullary nail

    B. Cerclage wire

    C. Semitubular plate

    D. Ilizarov device

28. Which of the following orthopedic devices is often used during a hip pinning?

    A. Cannulated screw assembly

    B. Ilizarov device

    C. Kirschner wire

    D. Semitubular plate

29. Which of the following devices is often used to reduce femoral, tibial, and humeral shaft fractures?

    A. Intramedullary nail

    B. Cerclage wire

    C. Ilizarov device

    D. Compression screw

30. What is the name of the newer type of prosthetic device to replace a defective hip joint?

    _____

31. A surgical procedure performed to alleviate pain caused by bony neural impingement involving the spine is termed

    _____ .

32. What is the name of the device used to stabilize the vertebral body in lieu of traditional spinal fusion?

    _____

19

33. In what position is the patient placed during most cervical laminectomies? _____

34. List the two internal fixators commonly used during scoliosis surgery:

A. _____   B. _____

35. Match each of the following surgical terms and devices to its correct definition:

_____ A. Orthopedic wire that tightens around fracture site to reduce shortening of limb

_____ B. Narrow, orthopedic screw designed to enter and fix cortical bone

_____ C. Large screw used in internal fixation of nondisplaced fractures of proximal femur

_____ D. Fabricated (artificial) substitute for a diseased or missing anatomic part

_____ E. Isolation drape that separates the sterile field from the nonsterile environment

_____ F. Soaking of moisture through a sterile or nonsterile drape, cover, or protective barrier

_____ G. Unthreaded (smooth) or threaded metallic wire used to reduce fractures of wrist (carpals) and individual bones of the hands and feet

_____ H. Orthopedic screw designed to enter and fix porous and spongy bone

_____ I. Creation of an artificial joint to correct ankylosis

_____ J. Electrohydraulic shock waves use to break apart calcifications in the urinary system

1. Arthroplasty
2. Cancellous screw
3. Cannulated screw
4. Cerclage wire
5. Cortical screw
6. ESWL
7. Kirschner wire
8. Prosthesis
9. Shower curtain
10. Strike through

Answers to Review Exercises

Review Exercise A: Radiographic Trauma and Fracture Terminology

1. True
2. True
3. False (It is important to rotate the x-ray tube and image receptor around patients if they are unable to move.)
4. A. Dislocation
   B. Luxation
5. A. Shoulder
   B. Fingers or thumb
   C. Patella
   D. Hip
6. Subluxation
7. Sprain
8. Contusion
9. Apposition
10. Bayonet apposition
11. A. Varus (deformity) angulation
    B. Lateral apex
12. A simple fracture does not break through the skin, but a compound fracture protrudes through the skin.
13. A. Torus fracture
    B. Greenstick fracture
14. Butterfly fracture
15. Impacted fracture
16. A. Chauffeur's
    B. Mallet
    C. Open
    D. Ping-pong
    E. Closed
17. False. (A chip fracture involves an isolated fracture not associated with a tendon or ligament.)
18. Closed reduction
19. 1. G
    2. H
    3. A
    4. I
    5. D
    6. J
    7. B
    8. M
    9. L
    10. N
    11. F
    12. O
    13. E
    14. K
    15. C
20. A. Colles' fracture
    B. Distal radius, posterior displacement of distal fragment
    C. Fall on outstretched arm
21. A. Pott's fracture
    B. Distal fibula and occasionally the distal tibia or medial malleolus

Review Exercise B: Positioning Principles and Grids

1. Adaptation
2. Move the CR and IR around the patient to produce similar projections rather than moving the patient.
3. Two. Two projections should be taken 90° to each other.
4. Two. Both joints must be included on the initial study.
5. False (must include at least one joint nearest injury)
6. 10
7. A. Correct CR centering
   B. Correct CR angling
   C. Correct grid focal range
8. True
9. False (parallel to)
10. The SID range in which the x-ray beam can pass through the grid without excessive absorption
11. 6:1 or 8:1 grid ratio
12. 34 to 46 inches (86 to 117 cm)
13. 48 to 72 inches (122 to 183 cm)
14. It will create "off-distance" grid cutoff.
15. True
16. B. 6:1 or 8:1

Review Exercise C: Mobile X-Ray Equipment and Radiation Protection

1. A. Battery-powered, battery-driven type
   B. Standard AC power source, nonmotor drive
2. Standard power source, nonmotor drive
3. 8 hours
4. True
5. C-arm
6. A. X-ray tube
   B. Image intensifier
7. Because it results in a significant increase in exposure to the head and neck region of the operator
8. A. Intensifier side
   B. The radiation field pattern extends out farther on the x-ray tube side.
9. Left monitor
10. True
11. True
12. False (reduces exposure to patient)
13. True
14. False (can be used)
15. Roadmapping
16. A. Draping the total C-arm, tube, and intensifier
    B. Draping the patient

C. Using a "shower curtain" type of arrangement to maintain a sterile field
17. A. Time
    B. Distance
    C. Shielding
18. Distance
19. C. Use intermittent or "foot-tapping" fluoroscopy
20. C. 50 to 100 mR/hr
21. A. 5 mR (60 mR ÷ 60 min = 1 mR × 5 min = 5)
22. B. 25 mR/hr
23. 67 mR (400 ÷ 60 x 10 = 67)
24. C. 100 to 300 mR/hr
25. Four

Review Exercise D: Trauma and Mobile Positioning and Procedures

1. Centered 3 to 4 inches (7 to 10 cm) below jugular notch, angled caudad so as to be perpendicular to sternum
2. False (not recommended because of probable grid cutoff)
3. A. Crosswise
   B. To prevent side cutoff of the right or left lateral margins of the chest. More important with portable chests because of increased divergence of x-ray beam at the shorter SID.
4. Right lateral decubitus
5. 15° to 20° LPO
6. Crosswise
7. 30° to 40° cross-angled mediolateral projection (NOTE: This results in image distortion and should be done as a last resort.)
8. A. Left lateral decubitus
9. D. Dorsal decubitus
10. Increased OID of the thumb (increases distortion)
11. PA and lateral projections
12. C. 65 kV and 10 mAs
13. True
14. True
15. AP and horizontal beam, transthoracic lateral or scapular "Y" projection
16. A horizontal beam transthoracic lateral
17. B. 15°
18. A. 20 to 30
19. C. 10° posteriorly from perpendicular to plantar surface (NOTE: This would also be 10° posteriorly from plane of IR.)

20. Angle the CR 15° to 20° lateromedially to the long axis of the foot.
21. AP and horizontal beam lateral with no flexion of knee
22. 45° lateromedial cross-angle AP projection of the knee and proximal tibia/fibula
23. A. Danelius-Miller method
24. Mediolateral (Sanderson) projection
25. Cross-angled mediolaterally to be near perpendicular to the long axis of the foot
26. Swimmer's lateral using a horizontal beam CR
27. D. 35° to 40° cephalad axial projection
28. 45° oblique using the double-angle method with IR perpendicular to CR
29. A. 45° medial
    B. 15° cephalad
30. Cassette is placed on a stool under the table, and patient is set at a 45° angle, perpendicular to CR.
31. C. Horizontal beam lateral skull
32. C. AP skull, CR 15° cephalad to OML
33. True
34. False (should not exceed 45°)
35. Parallel to the mentomeatal line, centered to acanthion
36. 25° to 30° cephalad and possibly 5° to 10° posterior to clear the shoulder
37. D. PA or AP and horizontal beam lateral forearm
38. A. Pediatric

39. A. AP and horizontal beam lateral lower leg
40. C. Stellate fracture

Review Exercise E: Surgical Radiography

1. A. Confidence
   B. Mastery
   C. Problem-solving skills
   D. Communication
2. A. 2
   B. 3
   C. 6
   D. 4
   E. 1
   F. 5
3. False
4. False
5. True
6. False
7. A. Drape the image intensifier, x-ray tube, and C-arm using a sterile cloth and/or bags.
   B. Drape the patient or surgery site with an additional sterile cloth before the undraped C-arm is positioned over the anatomy.
   C. Maintain the sterile area by using a "shower curtain."
8. Asepsis
9. C
10. D
11. False
12. True
13. True
14. False
15. Aerosol

16. Added patient dose
17. Brighter image
18. A
19. Biliary ductal system
20. "Pizza pan"
21. Crosswise to prevent grid cutoff
22. 6 to 8 ml
23. A. Can be performed as an outpatient procedure
    B. Less invasive procedure
    C. Reduced hospital time and cost
24. D
25. B
26. C
27. D
28. A
29. A
30. Modular bipolar hip prostheses
31. Laminectomy
32. Interbody fusion cages
33. Supine
34. A. Harrington rods
    B. Luque rods
35. A. 4
    B. 5
    C. 3
    D. 8
    E. 9
    F. 10
    G. 7
    H. 2
    I. 1
    J. 6

SELF-TEST

My Score = _____ %

Directions: This self-test should be taken only after completing all of the readings, review exercises, and laboratory activities for a particular section. The purpose of this test is not only to provide a good learning exercise but also to serve as a strong indicator of what your final evaluation exam will be. It is strongly suggested that if you do not get at least a 90% to 95% grade on this self-test, you review those areas in which you missed questions before going to your instructor for the final evaluation exam for this chapter. (There are 90 questions or blanks—each is worth 1.1 points.)

1. From the list of possible fracture types below, indicate which fracture is represented on each drawing or radiograph by writing in the correct term where indicated (*A* through *I*):

   • Single (closed) fracture

   • Compound (open) fracture

   • Torus fracture

   • Greenstick fracture

   • Plastic fracture

   • Transverse fracture

   • Oblique fracture

   • Spiral fracture

   • Comminuted fracture

   • Impacted fracture

   • Baseball (mallet) fracture

   • Barton's fracture

   • Bennett fracture

   • Colles' fracture

   • Monteggia's fracture

   • Nursemaid's elbow fracture

   • Pott's fracture

   • Avulsion fracture

   • Chip fracture

   • Compression fracture

   • Stellate fracture

   • Tuft fracture

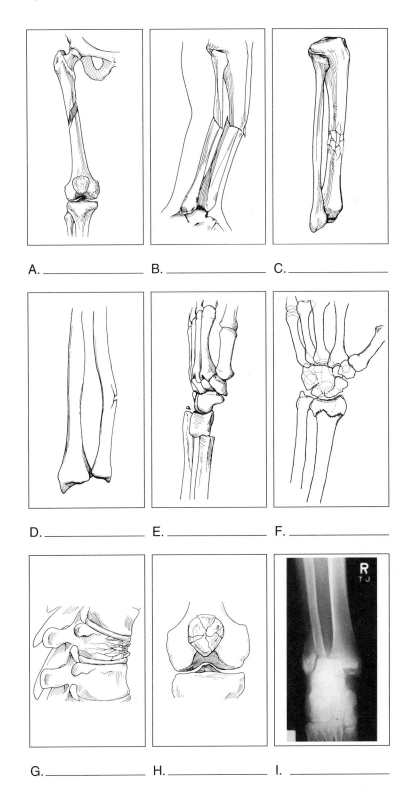

A. _____   B. _____   C. _____

D. _____   E. _____   F. _____

G. _____   H. _____   I. _____

2. A. What is the correct term for the displacement of a bone from a joint? _____

    B. What is the correct term for a partial displacement? _____

3. What region of the body encounters partial dislocations most frequently? _____

4. Which one of the following terms describes a poor alignment between the ends of a fractured bone?

    A. Dislocation   C. Apex angulation

    B. Lack of apposition   D. Anatomic apposition

5. Which one of the following terms describes a bending of a distal fracture away from the midline?

    A. Valgus angulation   C. Apex angulation

    B. Varus angulation   D. Bayonet apposition

6. Match each of the following types of fracture to its correct definition (using each answer only once):

    _____ A. Fracture through the pedicles of C2   1. Nursemaid's elbow

    _____ B. Fracture of proximal half of ulna with dislocation of radial head   2. Bennett's

    _____ C. Fracture due to a disease process   3. Baseball

    _____ D. Fracture resulting in an isolated bone fragment   4. Pathologic

    _____ E. Subluxation of the radial head on a child   5. Hangman's

    _____ F. Fracture along base of first metacarpal   6. Hutchinson's

    _____ G. Fracture of distal phalanx with finger extended   7. Stress or fatigue

    _____ H. Also called a *March fracture*   8. Chip

    _____ I. Also called a *Chauffeur's fracture*   9. Monteggia's

7. True/False: Any trauma study requires at least two projections as close to 90° opposite from each other as possible.

8. True/False: On an initial study of a long bone, both joints should be included for each projection.

9. Which one of the following projections (on a sthenic adult) would require the use of a grid?

    A. AP leg (tibia-fibula)   C. Lateral elbow

    B. Lateral ankle   D. AP shoulder

10. What is the preferred grid ratio for trauma radiography?

    A. 5:1   C. 10:1 to 12:1

    B. 6:1 to 8:1   D. 16:1

11. List the two factors that determine a grid's focal range:

    A. _____   B. _____

12. True/False: Using an SID greater than the established focal range will produce grid cutoff.

13.   Which type of mobile radiography x-ray unit is self-propelled? _____

14.   Which type of mobile x-ray unit is lighter-weight? _____

15.   True/False: C-arms are most generally stationary fluoroscopy units used in surgery.

16.   True/False: The C-arm fluoroscopy unit can be rotated a minimum of 180°.

17.   True/False: The AP projection with the x-ray tube placed directly above the anatomy during a C-arm procedure is recommended to minimize OID.

18.   True/False: Digital C-arm units can store images on video tape or computer hard disk memory.

19.   What is the term for the process of holding one image on the C-arm monitor while also providing continuous

      fluoroscopy? _____

20.   What is the primary benefit of the "pulse mode" on a digital C-arm unit? _____

21.   List the three cardinal rules of radiation protection:

      A.   _____   B.   _____   C.   _____

22.   Which one of the cardinal rules is most effective in reducing occupational exposure? _____

23.   **Situation:** A technologist using a C-arm fluoroscope receives 125 mR/hr standing 2 feet from the patient. What is the exposure rate if the technologist moves to a distance of 6 feet?

      A.   Less than 10 mR/hr   C.   30 to 50 mR/hr

      B.   15 to 30 mR/hr   D.   50 to 75 mR/hr

24.   **Situation:** A technologist receives 30 mR/hr during a C-arm fluoroscopic procedure. What is the *total* exposure

      dose if the procedure takes 8 minutes of fluoroscopy time? _____

25.   True/False: The exposure dose is greater on the image intensifier side than on the x-ray tube side with the C-arm in the horizontal configuration.

26.   True/False: A 30° tilt of C-arm from the vertical perspective will increase the dose by a factor of three to the head and neck region.

27.   **Situation:** A patient with a possible pleural effusion in the right lung enters the emergency room. The patient is unable to stand or sit erect. What position would best demonstrate this condition?

      A.   Right lateral decubitus   C.   Dorsal decubitus

      B.   AP supine   D.   Semierect AP

28.   Where is the CR centered for an AP semierect projection of the chest? _____

29.   **Situation:** A patient with a crushing injury to the thorax enters the emergency room. The patient is on a backboard and cannot be moved. Which projections can be performed to determine whether the sternum is fractured?

19

30. **Situation:** A patient with possible ascites enters the emergency room. The patient is unable to stand or sit erect. Which one of the following positions would best demonstrate this condition?

   A. AP supine KUB   C. Left lateral decubitus

   B. Dorsal decubitus   D. Prone KUB

31. How many projections are required for a postreduction study of the wrist? _____

32. How is the CR aligned for a trauma lateral projection of the elbow? _____

33. Which lateral projection would best demonstrate the mid-to-distal humerus without rotating the limb?

   _____

34. How much rotation of the body is generally required for a lateromedial scapula projection with a trauma patient

   who can be turned up partially on her side? _____

35. To ensure that the CR is aligned properly for an AP trauma projection of the foot, the CR is angled:

   _____

36. **Situation:** A patient with a possible fracture of the ankle enters the emergency room. The patient cannot rotate the lower limb. What can be done to provide the orthopedic surgeon with a mortise projection of the ankle?

   _____

37. Which one of the following statements is *not* true about the Sanderson method?

   A. The unaffected leg does not need to be moved at all.

   B. The patient is obliqued into a 15° to 20° posterior oblique position.

   C. The affected leg is rotated 10° to 15° internally if possible.

   D. The CR is angled to be perpendicular to the long axis of the foot of the affected limb.

38. Which one of the following projections will demonstrate the C1-2 vertebra if the patient cannot open his mouth?

   A. 35° to 40° cephalad, AP axial projection   C. 15° to 20° cephalad, AP axial projection

   B. Swimmer's lateral   D. Articular pillar projection

39. **Situation:** A patient with a possible fracture of the cervical spine pedicles enters the emergency room. Which one of the following projections will best demonstrate this region of the spine with the least distortion without moving the patient?

   A. Perform a swimmer's lateral

   B. Perform an articular pillar projection

   C. Perform a double-angle oblique projection with IR perpendicular to CR

   D. Perform a 45° CR oblique projection with IR flat on tabletop

40. What are the two advantages of angling the cassette 45° for the trauma oblique cervical, which also results in a long OID for the Method Two double-angle projection?

   A. _____   B. _____

41. Which one of the following facial bone projections will best demonstrate air-fluid levels in the maxillary sinuses for a patient unable to stand or sit erect?

    A. AP acanthioparietal   C. AP modified acanthioparietal

    B. Trauma, horizontal beam lateral D. AP axial

42. A. On a horizontal beam lateral trauma skull projection, should the IR be placed lengthwise or crosswise to the

        patient? _____

    B. Where should the CR be centered for this lateral skull projection? _____

43. **Situation:** A patient with a possible compression fracture of the lumbar spine enters the emergency room. Which specific position of the lumbar spine series would best demonstrate this fracture?

    A. AP   C. Lateral

    B. LPO and RPO   D. AP L5-S1 projection

44. **Situation:** A patient with a possible Barton's fracture comes to the radiology department. Which one of the following positioning routines would best demonstrate this?

    A. AP or PA and lateral wrist   C. AP and lateral foot

    B. AP, mortise, and lateral ankle   D. AP and lateral lower leg

45. Radiologists often use the Salter-Harris system to classify _____ fractures.

    A. Pathologic   C. Stellate

    B. Trimalleolar   D. Epiphyseal

46. **Situation:** A patient enters the ER with a possible radial head dislocation. The arm is immobilized with the elbow flexed 90°. Which one of the following projections will best demonstrate the radial head free of superimposition of the ulna without having to extend the elbow?

    A. AP partial flexion   C. Jones' method

    B. Trauma axiolateral projection   D. Lateromedial projection

47. For successful surgical radiographic exposures, clear communication must be established between the surgeon, technologist, and:

    A. Scrub   C. Circulator

    B. CST   D. Anesthesiologist

48. CST is the acronym for _____ .

49. Suctioning, tying, and clamping blood vessels, as well as assisting in cutting and suturing tissues, are the general duties of the:

    A. CST   C. Surgical assistant

    B. Circulator   D. Scrub

50. Which one of the following devices helps maintain the sterile environment in surgery during a C-arm guided hip pinning?

    A. Shower curtain   C. Cassette cover

    B. Mylar shield   D. Good cleaning of equipment before procedure

19

51. The absence of infectious organisms is the definition for:

   A. Surgical cleanliness   C. Asepsis

   B. Sepsis   D. Surgical sterility

52. What portion(s) of the OR table is(are) considered sterile:

   A. Only the level of the tabletop

   B. Entire table

   C. Tabletop and half of the base

   D. None of the table

53. True/False: Scrubs worn in radiology may be also worn in surgery.

54. True/False: Scrub covers must be removed before entering the surgical suite.

55. True/False: The technologist can wear nonsterile gloves when handling the IR and surgical cover following a procedure.

56. Imaging equipment permanently stored in surgery must be cleaned at least:

   A. Daily   C. Monthly

   B. Bimonthly   D. Weekly

57. Which one of the following techniques will best reduce dose to the surgical team during a C-arm procedure?

   A. Use boost function whenever possible.

   B. Place tube in vertical position above patient.

   C. Use intermittent fluoroscopy.

   D. Lower kV as low as possible.

58. **Situation:** An image taken during an operative cholangiogram reveals that the biliary ducts are superimposed over the spine. The surgeon wants the ducts projected away from the spine. Which one of the following positions may eliminate this problem during the repeat exposure?

   A. Shallow RPO   C. AP

   B. Shallow LPO   D. Horizontal beam lateral

59. True/False: Laparoscopic cholecystectomy is not suited for every patient and condition.

60. Retrograde urography is a _____ (**nonfunctional** or **functional**) examination of the urinary system.

61. A retrograde pyelogram is a specific radiographic examination of the _____ system.

62. ORIF is the abbreviation for _____ .

63. Which one of the following orthopedic devices is used to stabilize a midfemoral shaft fracture?

   A. Austin-Moore prosthesis   C. Interbody fusion cages

   B. Intramedullary rod   D. Cannulated screw

64.   Which one of the following devices is an example of an external fixator?

    A.   Interbody fusion cage   C.   Modular bipolar prosthesis

    B.   Thompson prosthesis   D.   Ilizarov device

65.   Which one of the following procedures does **not** require the use of mobile fluoroscopy?

    A.   Hip pinning   C.   Open reduction of tibia

    B.   Intramedullary rod insertion   D.   All of the above require fluoroscopic guidance

66.   Which of the following devices can be used for spinal fusion surgery rather than the use of a pedicle screw?

    A.   Austin-Moore prosthesis   C.   Dynamic compression plate

    B.   Cannulated screw   D.   Interbody fusion cage

67.   Which spinal procedure may require the use of Harrington or Luque rods?

    A.   Scoliosis corrective surgery   C.   Spinal fusion

    B.   Microdiscectomy   D.   All of the above

68.   An unthreaded (smooth) or threaded metallic wire used to reduce fractures of the wrist (carpals) is called

    _____ .

69.   A special OR table used for hip pinnings and other orthopedic procedures to provide traction to the involved limb

    is termed _____ .

70.   DHS is an abbreviation for _____ .

CHAPTER 20

Pediatric Radiography

Positioning considerations are unique to pediatric radiography and present a definite challenge for all technologists. Children cannot be handled and positioned like miniature adults. They have special needs and require patience and understanding. Their anatomic makeup is vastly different from that of adults, especially the skeletal system. The bony development (ossification) of children goes through specific growth stages from infancy to adolescence. These need to be understood by technologists so that the appearance of the normal growth stages can be recognized. Examples of normal bone development patterns at various ages are included in this chapter and in the textbook.

The basic and optional projections and positions are much different for children than for adults. You need to know and understand these differences to be able to visualize the essential anatomy on children of various ages.

The most obvious differences for children when compared with adults are the methods of positioning and immobility. Small children cannot just be instructed to hold still in certain positions or to hold their breath during the exposure. You will need to learn how to relate to children and communicate with them to get their cooperation without forceful immobilization.

Special immobilization techniques need to be learned along with the use of various types of commonly available immobilization paraphernalia. Specialized restraining devices available in many departments will be explained and demonstrated in this chapter.

Radiation protection for these small patients must also be a major concern, because the younger the child, the more sensitive the tissues are to radiation. Thus **accurate collimation and gonadal shielding** are absolutely essential. High-speed IR should also be used, and **repeats must be minimized.** Specific patient doses in icon boxes for each projection are not provided in this chapter because of the many variables involved. However, **keeping all child doses as low as possible** is even more important than in adult radiography. Therefore, careful study of this chapter and related clinical experience are essential **before** you attempt a radiographic examination on a small child or infant. As a student, you may have limited opportunity to observe and assist with pediatric patients during your training. This makes learning and mastering the information provided in this chapter of the textbook and this workbook–laboratory manual even more important.

CHAPTER OBJECTIVES

After you have successfully completed the activities in this chapter, you will be able to:

_____ 1. List the steps and process of the technologist's introduction to the child and parent and the potential role of the parent during the child's examination.

_____ 2. Define the term *nonaccidental trauma (NAT)* and describe the role of technologists if they suspect child abuse based on individual state guidelines.

_____ 3. Identify the more common commercial immobilization devices and explain their function.

_____ 4. List the most common types of ancillary devices used for immobilization.

_____ 5. List the six steps of "mummifying" an infant. Perform this procedure on a simulated patient.

_____ 6. Define terms relating to bone development or ossification and identify the radiographic appearance and the normal stages of development of secondary growth centers.

_____ 7. Identify methods of reducing patient and guardian doses and repeat exposures during pediatric procedures.

_____ 8. Identify alternative imaging modalities and procedures performed on pediatric patients.

_____ 9. List the common pathologic indications for radiographic examinations of the pediatric chest, upper and lower limbs, pelvis and hips, skull, and abdomen.

_____ 10. For select forms of pathology of the pediatric skeletal system, determine whether manual exposure factors would increase, decrease, or remain the same.

_____ 11. Describe positioning, technical factors, shielding requirements, and immobilization techniques for procedures of the chest, skeletal system, and abdomen.

_____ 12. List general patient preparation requirements for procedures of the pediatric abdomen, including specific minimum patient preparation requirements for the upper GI, lower GI, and IVU procedures.

_____ 13. List the types and quantities of contrast media based on age as recommended for upper GI, lower GI, and IVU procedures.

_____ 14. Using an articulated pediatric mannequin, correctly immobilize and position a patient. Using gonadal shielding, perform examinations of the chest, abdomen, upper limb, lower limb, pelvis and hips, and skull.

_____ 15. According to established evaluation criteria, critique and evaluate radiographs provided by your instructor for each of the previously mentioned examinations.

_____ 16. Discriminate between acceptable and unacceptable radiographs and describe how positioning or technical errors can be corrected.

20

Learning Exercises

The following review exercises should be completed only after careful study of the associated pages in the textbook as indicated by each exercise. Answers to each review exercise are given at the end of the review exercises.

Part I: Introduction to Pediatric Radiography

REVIEW EXERCISE A: Immobilization, Ossification, Radiation Protection, Preexam Preparation, and Pathologic Indications (see textbook pp. 654-663)

1. List the two important general factors that produce a successful pediatric radiographic procedure:

    A. _____

    B. _____

2. List the three possible roles for the parent during a pediatric procedure:

    A. _____

    B. _____

    C. _____

3. True/False: Parents should never be in the radiographic room with their child.

4. True/False: Battered child syndrome (BCS) is the acceptable term for child abuse.

5. True/False: The technologist is responsible for reporting potential signs of child abuse to the police.

6. True/False: The technologist should always use as short an exposure time as possible during pediatric procedures.

7. List the correct terms for the following descriptions of pediatric immobilization devices:

    A. A piece of Plexiglas with short Velcro straps for immobilization of upper and lower limbs: _____

    B. A device used to hold down upper or lower limbs without obscuring essential anatomy: _____

    C. A device with an adjustable-type bicycle seat and two clear plastic body clamps: _____

8. Which of the immobilization devices described in question 7 is most commonly used for erect chests and

    abdomens? _____

9.   True/False: Sandbags completely filled with fine sand should be used to immobilize pediatric patients.

10. If stockinettes are used for immobilization, what size should be used for a larger pediatric patient?

    A. 1 inch   C. 3 inch

    B. 2 inch   D. 4 inch

11. Which type of tape is *not* recommended for immobilization purposes on children (because it may create an artifact

    on the radiograph when placed over the region being radiographed)? _____

12. When adhesive tape is used to immobilize an infant (if not placed directly over parts to be radiographed), what two methods are used to prevent the adhesive tape from injuring the infant's fragile skin?

    A. _____

    B. _____

13. A. If Ace bandages are used for immobilization of the legs, which size should be used on infants and smaller

        children—3 inch, 4 inch, or 6 inch? _____

    B. What size should be used on older children? _____

14. Briefly describe the six steps for "mummifying" a child:

    A. _____

        _____

    B. _____

        _____

    C. _____

        _____

    D. _____

        _____

    E. _____

        _____

    F. _____

        _____

15. Primary centers of bone formation (ossification) involving the midshafts of long bones are called _____ .

16. Secondary centers of ossification of the long bones are called _____ .

17. The spaces between the primary and secondary areas of ossification are called _____ .

18. At approximately what age does the epiphysis of the fibular apex first become clearly visible? (see textbook, p. 658)

   A. 1 or 2 years old   C. 5 or 6 years old

   B. 3 or 4 years old   D. Teens

19. At approximately what age does the skeleton reach full ossification?

   A. 12 years old   C. 25 years old

   B. 18 years old   D. 40 years old

20. List three safeguards to help reduce repeat exposures during pediatric procedures:

   A. _____   C. _____

   B. _____

21. Other than gonadal shielding, what three safeguards can be used to reduce the patient dose during pediatric procedures?

   A. _____   C. _____

   B. _____

22. Sometimes a primary technologist and assisting technologist work together. Match each of the following duties with the correct technologist.

   _____ 1. Makes exposures   A. Primary technologist

   _____ 2. Positions the patient   B. Assisting technologist

   _____ 3. Processes the images

   _____ 4. Positions the tube and collimates

   _____ 5. Sets exposure factors

   _____ 6. Instructs the parents

23. True/False: Clothing, bandages, and diapers generally do not need to be removed from the regions being radiographed on pediatric patients since they do not cause artifacts on the radiographs (as long as metallic fasteners are not present).

24. Which one of the following imaging modalities is most effective in diagnosing pyloric stenosis in children?

   A. Sonography   C. Functional MRI

   B. Spiral/helical CT   D. Nuclear medicine

25. Functional MRI may be used to detect disorders in all the following conditions *except:*

   A. Autism   C. Hydrocephalus

   B. Tourette syndrome   D. Attention deficit hyperactivity disorder

26. Match each of the following pathologic indications of the pediatric chest with the best definition or description (using each choice only once):

    _____ A. Meconium aspiration   1. Bacterial infection can lead to closure of the upper airway

    _____ B. Hyaline membrane disease   2. Also known as *respiratory distress syndrome*

    _____ C. Neonate Graves' disease   3. Inherited disease leading to clogging of bronchi

    _____ D. Epiglottitis   4. May develop during stressful births

    _____ E. Cystic fibrosis   5. Viral infection leading to labored breathing and dry cough

    _____ F. Croup   6. Coughing up blood

    _____ G. Hemoptysis   7. A form of hyperthyroidism

27. Match each of the following pathologic indications of the pediatric skeletal system to the best definition or description:

    _____ A. Meningocele   1. Most common form of short-limbed dwarfism

    _____ B. Kohler's bone disease   2. Hereditary disorder characterized by soft and fragile bones

    _____ C. Legg-Calvé-Perthes disease   3. Congenital defect in which the spinal cord protrudes through an opening in the vertebral column

    _____ D. Talipes equinus
                                                4. A common lesion at the hip
    _____ E. Osteogenesis imperfecta
                                                5. Group of diseases affecting the epiphyseal plates of long bones
    _____ F. Achondroplasia
                                                6. Congenital defect in which the meninges of the spinal cord protrude through an opening in the vertebral column
    _____ G. Myelocele

    _____ H. Osteochondroses   7. Inflammation of the navicular bone in the foot

                                                8. Congenital deformity of the foot involving plantar flexion

28. Match each of the following pathologic indications of the pediatric abdomen to the best definition or description:

    _____ A. Hydronephrosis   1. May result in repeated, forceful vomiting

    _____ B. Pyloric stenosis   2. Characterized by absence of rhythmic contractions of large intestine

    _____ C. NEC   3. Condition characterized by absence of an opening in an organ

    _____ D. Atresias   4. Condition resulting from an allergic reaction to gluten

    _____ E. Hypospadias   5. Enlarged renal collection system due to obstruction

    _____ F. Hirschsprung's disease   6. Inflammation of the inner lining of the intestine

    _____ G. Celiac disease   7. Congenital defect in male urethra

29. Indicate whether the following pathologic conditions require that manual exposure factors be increased (+), be decreased (−), or remain the same (0):

    _____ A. Pneumonia

    _____ B. Pneumothorax

    _____ C. Osteogenesis imperfecta

    _____ D. Legg-Calvé-Perthes disease

    _____ E. Osteomalacia

    _____ F. Osteopetrosis

    _____ G. Volvulus

30. True/False: Malignant bone tumors are rare in young children.

Part II: Radiographic Positioning

REVIEW EXERCISE B: Pediatric Positioning of the Chest, Skeletal System, and Skull (see textbook pp. 665-676)

1. Complete the following technical factors for an AP or PA pediatric chest:

    A. Grid or nongrid? _____   D. SID, AP supine chest: _____

    B. kV range: _____   E. SID, PA erect chest: _____

    C. Image receptor—lengthwise or crosswise? _____

2. What kV range is generally used for a lateral chest? _____

3. Should a grid be used for a lateral chest? _____

4. The Pigg-O-Stat can be used effectively for an erect PA and lateral chest from infancy to approximately

    _____ years of age.

5. When should a chest exposure be made for a crying child?

    _____

6. Which radiographic structures are evaluated to determine rotation on a PA projection of the chest?

    _____

7. How is the x-ray tube aligned for a lateral projection of the chest if the patient is on a Tam-em board?

    _____

8. True/False: If available, the Pigg-O-Stat should be used rather than relying on parental assistance during a pediatric chest examination.

9. True/False: A well-inspired, erect chest radiograph taken on a young pediatric patient will visualize only six to seven ribs above the diaphragm.

10. True/False: The entire upper limb is commonly included on an infant rather than individual exposures of specific parts of the upper limb.

11. True/False: Except for survey exams, individual projections of the elbow, wrist, and shoulder should generally be taken on older children rather than including these regions on a single projection.

12. Match the following pathologic indicators with the correct radiographic procedure:

    _____ A. Atelectasis   1. Chest

    _____ B. Kohler's disease   2. Upper or lower limb

    _____ C. Cystic fibrosis

    _____ D. Talipes

    _____ E. RDS

13. Which single radiographic position will provide a lateral projection of bilateral lower limbs for the nontraumatic

    pediatric patient? _____

14. Which radiographic projections (and method) are performed for the infant with congenital club feet?

    _____

15. True/False: It is important to place the foot into true AP and lateral positions when performing a clubfoot study.

16. True/False: It is possible to provide gonadal shielding for both male and female pediatric patients for AP and lateral projections of hips.

17. What size image receptor should be used for a skull routine on a 6-year-old patient? _____

18. Which one of the following CR angulations will place the petrous ridges in the lower one-third of the orbits with an AP reverse Caldwell projection of the skull?

    A. 15° cephalad to OML   C. CR perpendicular to OML
    B. 15° caudad to OML   D. 30° cephalad to OML

19. Which one of the following pathologic indicators would apply to a pediatric skull series?

    A. Osteomyelitis   C. Mastoiditis
    B. CHD   D. Hyaline membrane disease

20. Which skull positioning line is placed perpendicular to the film for an AP Towne 30° caudal projection of the skull?

    A. IOML   C. MML
    B. OML   D. AML

21. True/False: Parental assistance for skull radiography is preferred rather than using head clamps and a mummy wrap on a pediatric patient.

22. True/False: Children over 5 years of age can usually hold their breath after a practice session.

23. Correct centering for the following can be achieved by placing the central ray at the level of which structure or landmark?

    A. AP, PA, or lateral chest: _____

    B. AP abdomen (infants and small children): _____

    C. AP supine abdomen (older children): _____

    D. AP skull: _____

REVIEW EXERCISE C: Positioning of the Pediatric Abdomen and Contrast Media Procedures (see textbook pp. 677-686)

1. True/False: The chest and abdomen are generally almost equal in circumference in the newborn.

2. True/False: Bony landmarks in infants are easy to palpate and locate.

3. True/False: It is difficult to distinguish the small bowel from the large bowel on a plain abdomen on an infant.

4. True/False: The radiographic contrast on a pediatric abdominal radiograph is high compared with that of an adult abdominal radiograph.

5. Complete the recommended NPO fasting before the following pediatric contrast media procedures:

    A. Infant to 1-year-old upper GI: _____   C. Infant lower GI: _____

    B. 1 year and older upper GI: _____   D. Pediatric IVU: _____

6. List five conditions that contraindicate the use of laxatives or enemas in preparation for a lower GI study:

    A. _____

    B. _____

    C. _____

    D. _____

    E. _____

7. Place an X next to the pathologic indicators that apply for an AP abdomen (KUB).

    _____ A. Croup   _____ E. Mastoiditis

    _____ B. NEC   _____ F. Hepatomegaly

    _____ C. Intussusception   _____ G. Appendicitis

    _____ D. Foreign body localization   _____ H. Hydrocephalus

8. Where is the CR centered for an erect abdomen on a small child? _____

9. A. What is the minimum kV for an AP abdomen projection of a newborn without a grid? _____

   B. A grid is recommended for a pediatric AP abdomen if the abdomen measures more than _____ cm.

10. Which one of the following projections of the abdomen will best demonstrate the prevertebral region?

    A. AP supine KUB   B. PA prone KUB   C. Dorsal decubitus abdomen   D. AP erect abdomen

11. Which one of the following conditions is caused by inflammation of the inner lining of the large or small bowel, resulting in tissue death?

    A. NEC   B. CHD   C. Intussusception   D. Meconium ileus

12. Which of the following procedures or projections should be performed for a possible meconium ileus?

    A. IVU procedure   B. Barium enema   C. AP supine abdomen   D. AP erect abdomen

13. How much barium should be given to each of the following patients for an upper GI series?

    A. Newborn to 1 year old: _____   C. 3 to 10 years old: _____

    B. 1 to 3 years old: _____   D. Over 10 years old: _____

14. What is the only recourse if a pediatric patient refuses to drink barium for an upper GI series?

    _____

15. True/False: A piece of lead vinyl should be placed beneath the child's lower pelvis during conventional fluoroscopy to reduce the gonadal/mean bone marrow dose.

16. True/False: The transit time of the contrast media for reaching the cecum during a pediatric small bowel series is approximately 2 hours.

17. True/False: Latex enema tips should be used for barium enemas for children under the age of 1 year.

18. True/False: Small retention enema tips can be used on infants during a barium enema to help barium retention.

19. What type of contrast media is recommended for reducing an intussusception? _____

20. What is the maximum height of the barium enema bag before the beginning of the procedure? _____

21. A backward flow of urine from the bladder into the ureters and kidneys is called _____ .

22. A malignant tumor of the kidney common in children under the age of 5 years is:

    A. Wilms' tumor   B. Adenocarcinoma   C. Ewing's sarcoma   D. Teratoma

23. What is the most common pathologic indication for a voiding cystourethrogram? _____

24. True/False: A radionuclide study for vesicourethral reflux provides a smaller patient dose compared to a fluoroscopic voiding cystourethrogram.

25. Indicate the suggested contrast media dosages for IVU procedures for each of the following weight categories of pediatric patients:

    A. 0 to 12 lb: _____

    B. 13 to 25 lb: _____

    C. 26 to 50 lb: _____

    D. 51 to 100 lb: _____

    E. >100 lb: _____

20

26. Identify the suggested contrast media dosages for each of the following metric weight measurements:

    A.   0 to 11 kg: _____

    B.   12 to 23 kg: _____

    C.   24 to 45 kg: _____

    D.   >45 kg: _____

27. True/False: The lower abdomen can be shielded for the 3-minute film taken during an IVU for both males and females.

28. True/False: To help depress the large bowel and create a radiolucent window to better visualize the kidneys, a carbonated drink should be given to pediatric patients before an IVU.

29. True/False: Most radiologists prefer their pediatric patients to be dehydrated before an IVU.

30. True/False: Since allergic reactions to iodinated contrast agents are rare in pediatric patients, the use of ionic contrast media is recommended for IVUs.

REVIEW EXERCISE D: Problem Solving and Analysis

1. **Situation:** A young child is sent to the radiology department for a skull series. The guardian states that she is willing to hold her child during the exposures; however, the guardian is 8 months pregnant. What should the technologist do next?

   A.   Place a 0.5-mm lead apron on the guardian and allow her to hold her child.

   B.   The technologist should hold the child during each exposure and have the guardian wait outside.

   C.   Have another health professional (nonradiology) hold the child and have the guardian wait outside the room.

   D.   Have a radiography student hold the child and have the guardian wait outside of the room.

2. **Situation:** A 3-year-old child comes to the radiology department for an erect abdomen examination. He is unable to hold still for the exposures. Which immobilization device should be used for this patient?

   A.   Tam-em board   C.   Plexiglas hold-down paddle

   B.   Pigg-O-Stat   D.   Compression or retention bands

3. **Situation:** A child comes to the radiology department with possible croup. Which one of the following procedures will best demonstrate this condition?

   A.   AP and lateral upper airway   C.   PA and lateral chest

   B.   Erect abdomen   D.   Sinus series

4. **Situation:** A newborn is diagnosed with RDS. Which one of the following procedures is commonly performed for this condition?

   A.   Abdomen   C.   CT of head

   B.   Functional MRI   D.   Chest

5. **Situation:** A child comes to the radiology department with a clinical history of Legg-Calvé-Perthes disease. Which one of the following projections will best demonstrate this condition?

   A.   PA and lateral chest   C.   AP and lateral hip

   B.   Supine and erect abdomen   D.   AP and lateral bilateral lower limbs

6. **Situation:** A child comes to the radiology department with a clinical history of Kohler's bone disease. Which one of the following radiographic routines will demonstrate this condition?

   A.   Foot   C.   Lumbar spine

   B.   Shoulder   D.   Cervical spine

7. **Situation:** A child comes to radiology with a clinical history of talipes equinus. Which of the following positioning routines/methods is often performed for this condition?

    A. Coyle method   C. AP and lateral foot—Kite method

    B. Erect AP knee projections   D. AP and lateral hip

8. **Situation:** Which radiographic procedure is often performed for Hirschsprung's disease?

    A. Upper GI   C. IVU

    B. MRI   D. Barium enema

9. **Situation:** Which radiographic procedure is often performed for pyloric stenosis?

    A. Barium enema   C. Enteroclysis

    B. Evacuative proctography   D. Upper GI

10. Which one of the following modalities is effective in detecting signs of autism?

    A. fMRI   C. Spiral CT

    B. Ultrasound   D. Nuclear medicine

20

Part III: Laboratory Exercises (see textbook pp. 655-676)

Exercises A and B need to be carried out in a radiographic laboratory or a general diagnostic room in the radiology department. General immobilization paraphernalia must be available (i.e., tape, sheets or large towels, sandbags, various sizes and shapes of positioning sponge blocks, retention bands, head clamps, stockinettes, and Ace bandages). More common commercial immobilization devices such as the Tam-em board or the Pigg-O-Stat (or similar devices) are optional if available. At least one of these devices should be made available for student use.

    Exercise C can be carried out in a classroom or any room in which illuminators (view boxes) are available.

LABORATORY EXERCISE A: Immobilization

For this section you will need some type of large articulated doll/mannequin to use as your patient. The doll should have arms and legs that are flexible (similar to those of a child). This does not need to be a phantom-like doll since radiographs will not be taken, but it will be used to simulate immobilization techniques and positioning for various body parts.

Check off each of the following activities as you complete them:

_____ 1. Complete the six steps of "mummifying."

_____ 2. Use a tubular-type stockinette of appropriate size to immobilize the "patient's" arms with hands placed above and behind the head.

_____ 3. Use the appropriate size Ace bandage to immobilize the lower limbs by wrapping with appropriate tension from the hips to the ankles.

_____ 4. Apply a retention band correctly across the abdomen and upper and lower limbs to completely immobilize these parts of the "patient."

_____ 5. Use sandbags under and over the legs and over each arm to immobilize for an AP abdomen.

_____ 6. Apply tape correctly in combination with sandbags to immobilize the head and the upper and lower limbs.

_____ 7. Apply head clamps to immobilize the head in combination with mummification of the patient and the use of sandbags or a retention band to prevent limb or body movement.

Tam-em board (if available):

_____   8.   Immobilize your patient correctly with the Velcro straps to restrain the upper and lower limbs and across the pelvic region.

Pigg-O-Stat (if available):

_____   9.   Immobilize your patient correctly with the arms above the head using the plastic side body clamps to restrain the arms and head.

LABORATORY EXERCISE B: Physical Positioning

This section again requires the use of a large articulated pediatric mannequin. Practice the following projections or positions until you can perform them accurately and without hesitation. Place a check mark by each activity when you have achieved it.

Include the details listed below as you simulate the basic projections for each exam that follows. Assume that the patient will not cooperate and that forceful immobilization is required. Use suggested immobilization techniques.

_____   Correct size and type of image receptor (appropriate for size of "patient")

_____   Correct centering of part to image receptor

_____   Correct SID and location and angle of central ray

_____   Selection of appropriate restraining devices and application of the same

_____   Correct placement of markers

_____   Correct use of contact gonadal shield

_____   Accurate collimation to body part of interest

_____   Approximate correct exposure factors

EXAMINATION	_IMMOBILIZATION_
_____ 1. AP chest, supine	Tam-em board or sandbags and/or stockinette and "Ace" bandages
_____ 2. Lateral chest, patient recumbent in lateral position	Sandbags and tape; or retention band

If Tam-em board is available:

_____ 3. Lateral chest, patient supine, horizontal beam CR	Tam-em board (see textbook, p. 655)

If Pigg-O-Stat is available:

_____	4.	PA chest erect, 72-inch (180-cm) SID	Pigg-O-Stat (see textbook, p. 655)
_____	5.	Lateral chest erect, 72-inch (180-cm) SID	Pigg-O-Stat (see textbook, p. 655)
_____	6.	AP abdomen, erect	Pigg-O-Stat (see textbook, p. 655)
_____	7.	AP abdomen, supine	Tam-em board; or tape, sandbags, and retention band (see textbook, p. 655)
_____	8.	AP and lateral upper limb (from shoulder to hand)	Tape, sandbags, and/or retention band (see textbook, p. 656)
_____	9.	AP and lateral lower limb (from hips to feet)	Tape, sandbags, and/or retention band (see textbook, p. 656)
_____	10.	AP and lateral feet (such as follow-up exams for clubfeet)	Sitting on pad using tape (see textbook, p. 656)
_____	11.	AP pelvis and hips	Tape and sandbags and/or retention band (see textbook, p. 656)
_____	12.	Lateral hips	Tape and sandbags and/or retention band (see textbook, p. 656)
_____	13.	AP skull, 15° AP and 30° Towne	Head clamps or tape for head. Mummification and sandbags or retention band for limbs and body (see textbook, p. 657)
_____	14.	Lateral skull, turned into lateral position	Head clamps or tape for head. Mummification and sandbags or retention band for limbs and body (see textbook, p. 657)
_____	15.	Lateral skull, horizontal beam in supine position	Tam-em board and tape for head (see textbook, p. 657)

LABORATORY EXERCISE C: Anatomy Review and Critique Radiographs of the Abdomen

Use the radiographs provided by your instructor. These should include optimal-quality and less-than-optimal quality radiographs of each of the following: chest, supine and erect abdomen, AP and lateral upper limb, AP and lateral pelvis and hips, AP and lateral lower limb, and AP and lateral skull radiographs.

Radiographs of the pelvis and upper and lower limbs of patients of various ages should be included to demonstrate the normal ossification or growth stages from infancy to adolescence.

Place a check mark by each of the following steps when completed:

_____ 1. Examine normal stages of growth by the appearance of the epiphyses in the pelvis and the long bones of the upper and lower limbs. Estimate the approximate age of the patient by the appearance of such epiphyses.

_____ 2. Critique each radiograph based on evaluation criteria provided for each projection in the textbook. Pediatric radiographs require a wider range of acceptable positioning criteria than for adults. Part centering and specific central ray locations are not as critical for pediatric radiographs because multiple anatomic parts or bones are included on one film. This is possible because detailed views of joint areas are not as important since these secondary growth areas are not yet fully developed. Thus complete limbs can be included on one film.

The following criteria guidelines can be used and checked as each radiograph is evaluated. Determine the corrections or adjustments in positioning or exposure factors necessary to bring those less-than-optimal radiographs up to a more desirable standard.

		RADIOGRAPHS					CRITERIA GUIDELINES
1	2	3	4	5	6		
___	___	___	___	___	___		a. Correct image receptor size as appropriate for age and size of patient?
___	___	___	___	___	___		b. Correct orientation of part to image receptor?
___	___	___	___	___	___		c. Acceptable alignment and/or centering of part to image receptor?
___	___	___	___	___	___		d. Correct collimation and correct CR angle where appropriate (such as for an AP skull)?
___	___	___	___	___	___		e. Evidence of gonadal shield correctly placed (if this should be visible)?
___	___	___	___	___	___		f. Pertinent anatomy well visualized?
___	___	___	___	___	___		g. Evidence of motion?
___	___	___	___	___	___		h. Optimal exposure (density and/or contrast)?
___	___	___	___	___	___		i. Patient ID with date and side markers visible without superimposing essential anatomy?

Answers to Review Exercises

Review Exercise A: Introduction, Immobilization, Ossification, Radiation Protection, Preexam Preparation, and Pathologic Indications

1. A. Technologist's attitude and approach to a child
   B. Technical preparation of the room
2. A. Serve as an observer in the room to lend support and comfort to their child
   B. Serve as a participator to assist with immobilization
   C. Remain in the waiting room, and do not accompany the child into the room
3. False (may be permissible with proper lead shielding if not pregnant)
4. False (correct term is *nonaccidental trauma, NAT*)
5. False (should report to radiologist or superior)
6. True
7. A. Tam-em board
   B. Plexiglas hold-down paddle
   C. Pigg-O-Stat
8. Pigg-O-Stat
9. False (should not be overfilled; should be soft and pliable)
10. D. 4 inch
11. Adhesive
12. A. Twisting the tape so that the adhesive surface is not against the skin
    B. Placing a gauze pad between the tape and the skin
13. A. 4 inch
    B. 6 inch
14. A. Place the sheet on the table folded in half or thirds lengthwise.
    B. Place patient in middle of sheet with the right arm down to the side. Fold sheet across the patient's body and pull sheet across the body, keeping the arm against the body.
    C. Place the patient's left arm along the side of the body and on top of the sheet. Bring the free sheet over the left arm to the right side of the body. Wrap the sheet around the body as needed.
    D. Pull the sheet tightly so that the patient cannot free arms.
    E. Place a long piece of tape from the right to the left wrapped arm

to prevent the patient from breaking out of the sheet.
    F. Place a piece of tape around the patient's knees.
15. Diaphysis
16. Epiphyses
17. Epiphyseal plates
18. C. 5 or 6 years old
19. C. 25 years old
20. A. Proper immobilization
    B. Short exposure times
    C. Accurate technique charts
21. A. Close collimation
    B. Low-dosage techniques
    C. Minimum number of images
22. 1. B, 2. A, 3. B, 4. A, 5. B, 6. A
23. False (These items may cause artifacts and should be removed.)
24. A. Sonography
25. C. Hydrocephalus
26. A. 4
    B. 2
    C. 7
    D. 1
    E. 3
    F. 5
    G. 6
27. A. 6
    B. 7
    C. 4
    D. 8
    E. 2
    F. 1
    G. 3
    H. 5
28. A. 5
    B. 1
    C. 6
    D. 3
    E. 7
    F. 2
    G. 4
29. A. (+)
    B. (−)
    C. (−)
    D. (0)
    E. (−)
    F. (+)
    G. (−)
30. True

Review Exercise B: Pediatric Positioning of the Chest, Skeletal System, and Skull

1. A. Nongrid
   B. 70 to 80 kV
   C. Crosswise
   D. 50 to 60 inches (127 to 212 cm)
   E. 72 inches (180 cm)

2. 75 to 80 kV
3. No
4. Two
5. As the child fully inhales and holds his or her breath
6. The sternoclavicular joints and lateral rib margins should be equidistant from the vertebral column.
7. Horizontally
8. True
9. False (9 or 10)
10. True
11. True
12. A. 1
    B. 2
    C. 1
    D. 2
    E. 1
13. Bilateral frog-leg
14. AP and lateral feet, Kite method
15. False (Take two projections 90° from each other.)
16. True (if correctly placed)
17. 10 × 12 inches (24 × 30 cm)—a child's skull is near adult size
18. A. 15° cephalad to OML
19. C. Mastoiditis
20. B. OML
21. False
22. True
23. A. Mamillary (nipple) line
    B. 1 inch (2.5 cm) above umbilicus
    C. At level of iliac crest
    D. Glabella

Review Exercise C: Positioning of the Pediatric Abdomen and Contrast Media Procedures

1. True
2. False (Most bony landmarks are nonexistent in infants.)
3. True
4. False (Contrast is low.)
5. A. 4 hours
   B. 6 hours
   C. No prep required
   D. 4 hours
6. A. Hirschsprung's disease
   B. Extensive diarrhea
   C. Appendicitis
   D. Obstruction
   E. Dehydration (patients who cannot withstand fluid loss)
7. The following indicators apply: B, C, D, F, G
8. 1 inch (2.5 cm) above the umbilicus
9. A. 65
   B. 10 cm
10. C. Dorsal decubitus abdomen

11. A. NEC
12. D. AP erect abdomen
13. A. 2 to 4 ounces
    B. 4 to 6 ounces
    C. 6 to 12 ounces
    D. 12 to 16 ounces
14. Insert a nasogastric tube into the stomach.
15. True
16. False (usually 1 hour)
17. False (Latex tips should not be used because of possible allergic response to latex.)
18. False (Retention tips should not be used on small children.)
19. Air for the pneumatic reduction of intussusception
20. 3 feet (for pediatric patients)
21. Vesicoureteral reflux

22. A. Wilms' tumor
23. Urinary tract infection (UTI)
24. True
25. A. 2 ml/lb
    B. 25 ml
    C. 1 ml/lb
    D. 50 ml
    E. ½ ml/lb
26. A. 3 ml/kg
    B. 2 ml/kg
    C. 50 ml
    D. 1 ml/kg
27. True
28. False (not recommended by pediatric radiologists)
29. False (should *not* be dehydrated)
30. False (nonionic types are recommended)

Review Exercise D: Problem Solving and Analysis

1. C. Have another health professional (nonradiology) hold the child and have the guardian wait outside of the room.
2. B. Pigg-O-Stat
3. A. AP and lateral upper airway
4. D. Chest
5. C. AP and lateral hip
6. A. Foot
7. C. Kite method
8. D. Barium enema
9. D. Upper GI
10. A. fMRI

SELF-TEST

My Score = _____ %

Directions: This self-test should be taken only after completing all of the readings, review exercises, and laboratory activities for a particular section. The purpose of this test is not only to provide a good learning exercise but also to serve as a good indicator of what your final evaluation exam will be. It is strongly suggested that if you do not get at least a 90% to 95% grade on this self-test, you review those areas where you missed questions before going to your instructor for the final evaluation exam for this chapter. (There are 78 questions or blanks—each is worth 1.3 points.)

1. At what age can most children be talked through a radiographic examination without forceful immobilization?

    A. 1 year   C. 3 years

    B. 2 years   D. 5 years

2. At the first meeting between the technologist and the patient (accompanied by an adult), which of the following generally should *not* be done?

    A. Introduce yourself

    B. Take the necessary time to explain what you will be doing

    C. Discuss the possible forceful immobilization that will be needed if the child will not cooperate

    D. Describe the total amount of radiation the patient will receive with that specific exam if it has to be repeated because of a lack of cooperation

    E. All of the above should be done

3. If child abuse is suspected by the technologist, he or she should:

    A. Ask the parent when the abuse occurred

    B. Report the abuse immediately to the necessary state officials as required by the state

    C. Refuse to do the examination or to touch the child until a physician has examined the patient

    D. Do none of the above

4. Which of the following is *not* the name of a known commercially available immobilization device?

    A. Posi-Tot   C. Pigg-O-Stat

    B. Tam-em board   D. Hold-em Tiger

5. The most suitable immobilization device for erect chests and/or the abdomen is the:

    A. Posi-Tot   C. Pigg-O-Stat

    B. Tam-em board   D. Hold-em Tiger

6. List the three factors that will reduce the number of repeat exposures with pediatric patients:

    A. _____   C. _____

    B. _____

7. What important question should a female parent be asked before allowing her to assist with holding her child

    during an exposure? _____

20

8. Which immobilization device or method should be used for an erect 1-year-old chest procedure? Assume these devices are available.

   A. Tam-em board   C. Pigg-O-Stat

   B. Hold-down paddle   D. Parent holding child

9. Which one of the following procedures can be performed to diagnose possible genetic fetal abnormalities?

   A. Nuclear medicine fetal scan   C. Functional MRI

   B. Spiral/helical CT   D. 3-D ultrasound

10. Which of the following procedures can be performed to evaluate children for attention deficient hyperactivity disorder?

    A. Spiral/helical CT   C. 3-D ultrasound

    B. Functional MRI   D. Nuclear medicine

11. Match each of the following conditions to its correct definition or statement (using each choice only once):

    _____ A. Croup

    _____ B. Respiratory distress syndrome

    _____ C. Epiglottitis

    _____ D. Osteochondroses

    _____ E. Osteogenesis imperfecta

    _____ F. Hydrocephalus

    _____ G. Osteomalacia

    _____ H. Hirschsprung's disease

    _____ I. Celiac disease

    _____ J. Neuroblastoma

    _____ K. Pyelonephritis

    _____ L. Atresia

    _____ M. Hepatomegaly

    1. Caused by an allergic reaction to gluten

    2. Group of diseases affecting the epiphyscal growth plates

    3. Abnormally enlarged ventricles in brain

    4. A common condition in children between the ages of 1 to 3, caused by a viral infection

    5. Enlargement of the liver

    6. Second-most common form of cancer in children under 5 years of age

    7. Bacterial infection of the upper airway that may be fatal if untreated

    8. Congenital defect in which an opening into an organ is missing

    9. Condition in which the alveoli and capillaries of the lungs are injured or infected

    10. Bacterial infection of the kidney

    11. Also known as *congenital megacolon*

    12. Also known as *rickets*

    13. Inherited condition that produces very fragile bones

12. Indicate whether the following pathologic conditions require that manual exposure factors be increased (+), be decreased (−), or remain the same (0):

    _____ A. Cystic fibrosis

    _____ B. Hyaline membrane disease

    _____ C. Osteogenesis imperfecta

    _____ D. Hydrocephalus

    _____ E. Idiopathic juvenile osteoporosis

    _____ F. Osteopetrosis

    _____ G. Volvulus

13. Which one of the following techniques will help remove the scapulae from the lung fields during chest radiography?

    A. Make exposure on the second inspiration   C. Extend arms upward

    B. Extend the chin   D. Place arms behind the patient's back

14. What is the typical kV range for a pediatric study of the upper limb? _____

15. True/False: A hand routine for a 7-year-old would be the same as for an adult patient.

16. True/False: For a bone survey of a young child, both limbs are commonly radiographed for comparison.

17. Which technique or method is performed to radiographically study congenital clubfoot? _____

18. Where is gonadal shielding placed for a bilateral hip study on a female pediatric patient?

    _____

19. Complete the following related to ossification by matching the correct term with the description. More than one choice per blank may be used.

    E = Epiphysis, D = Diaphysis, EP = Epiphyseal plate

    _____ 1. Primary centers

    _____ 2. Secondary centers

    _____ 3. Space between primary and secondary centers

    _____ 4. Occurs before birth

    _____ 5. Continues to change from birth to maturity

20. Match the following examinations with the pathologic indicators they are most likely associated with (answers may be used more than once):

_____ A. Intussusception   1. Chest

_____ B. NEC   2. Abdomen

_____ C. Hydrocephalus   3. Upper and lower limbs

_____ D. Atelectasis   4. Pelvis and hips

_____ E. Premature closure of fontanelles   5. Skull

_____ F. CHD

_____ G. Cystic fibrosis

_____ H. Meconium ileus

_____ I. Legg-Calvé-Perthes disease

_____ J. Hemoptysis

_____ K. Shunt check

_____ L. Bronchiectasis

_____ M. Hyaline membrane disease

21. How much is the CR angled from the OML for an AP Towne projection of the skull?

A. 15°   C. 25°

B. None   D. 30°

22. Where is the CR centered for a lateral projection of the pediatric skull?

A. At the EAM   C. 1 inch (2.5 cm) above the EAM

B. Midway between the glabella and inion   D. ¾ inch (2 cm) anterior and superior to the EAM

23. The NPO fasting period for a 6-month-old before an upper GI is:

A. 4 hours   C. 1 hour

B. 6 hours   D. 8 hours

24. Other than preventing artifacts in the bowel, what is the other reason that solid food is withheld for 4 hours before a pediatric IVU? _____

25. Which one of the following conditions would contraindicate the use of laxatives before a contrast media procedure?

A. Gastritis   C. Appendicitis

B. Blood in stool   D. Diverticulosis

26. Where is the CR centered for a KUB on:

A. An 8-year-old child? _____

B. A 1-year-old child? _____

27. At what level is the CR centered for a PA and lateral pediatric chest? _____

28. What is the recommended amount of barium for an 8-year-old child having an upper GI? _____

29. How is barium instilled into the large bowel for a barium enema study on an infant?

_____

30. What is the bowel prep for a pediatric voiding cystourethrogram (VCUG)? _____

31. When is urinary reflux most likely to occur during a VCUG? _____

32. For a pediatric small bowel study, the barium normally reaches the ileocecal region in _____ hour(s).

33. A VCUG on a child is most commonly performed to evaluate for (A) _____ and is

    generally scheduled to be completed (B) _____ (**before** or **after**) an IVU or ultrasound

    study of the kidneys.

34. True/False: Gonadal shielding should only be used in supine positions because of the difficulty in keeping the shield in place.

35. True/False: There should be no attempt to straighten out the abnormal alignment of the foot during a clubfoot study.

36. **Situation:** Which radiographic procedure is commonly performed for epiglottitis?

    A. Sinus series   C. CT of the chest

    B. AP and lateral upper airway   D. Functional MRI

37. **Situation:** Which of the following radiographic routines/procedures will best demonstrate Osgood-Schlatter disease?

    A. Barium enema   C. Upper GI

    B. AP and lateral hip   D. AP and lateral knee

38. **Situation:** A 2-year-old child comes to the radiology department for a routine chest examination. While removing the child's shirt, you notice a human bite mark on the upper arm. What should you do next?

    A. Call hospital security   C. Interview the parents about the injury

    B. Inform supervisor or physician D. Interview the child about the injury

39. Which of the following conditions can be diagnosed prenatally with sonography?

    A. Tourette syndrome   C. Spina bifida

    B. Vesicoureteral reflux   D. Autism

40. Which of the following imaging modalities is effective in detecting signs of attention deficit hyperactivity disorder (ADHD)?

    A. CT   C. Nuclear medicine

    B. Sonography   D. Functional MRI

CHAPTER 21

Angiography and Interventional Procedures

This chapter, which includes extensive detailed and somewhat complex anatomy and procedural information, is an excellent introduction to angiography and interventional procedures. It provides effective preparation and a good overview for the additional clinical training and experience that a cardiovascular technologist will need.

CHAPTER OBJECTIVES

After you have successfully completed the activities of this chapter, you will be able to:

_____ 1. List the divisions and components of the circulatory system.

_____ 2. List the three functions of the cardiovascular system.

_____ 3. On drawings, identify the components of the pulmonary and general systemic circulation.

_____ 4. Identify the four chambers of the heart, associated valves, and coronary circulation.

_____ 5. List and identify the four arteries supplying blood to the brain and the three branches arising from the aortic arch.

_____ 6. List the major branches of the external and internal carotid arteries and the primary divisions of the brain supplied by each.

_____ 7. On drawings, identify the major veins of the neck draining blood from the head and neck region.

_____ 8. List the major venous sinuses found in the cranium.

_____ 9. List the four segments of the thoracic aorta and describe the three common variations of the aortic arch.

_____ 10. List and identify the five major branches of the abdominal aorta.

_____ 11. List and identify the major abdominal veins.

_____ 12. List and identify the major arteries and veins of the upper and lower limbs.

_____ 13. List four functions of the lymphatic portion of the circulatory system.

_____ 14. Identify the six steps for the Seldinger technique

_____ 15. Identify the equipment generally found in a angiographic room.

_____ 16. Identify the pathologic indications, contraindications, and general procedure for cerebral angiography.

_____ 17. Identify the indications, catheterization technique, and general procedure for thoracic and abdominal angiography.

_____ 18. Identify the pathologic indications, contraindications, and general procedure for peripheral angiography.

_____ 19. Identify specific examples of vascular and nonvascular interventional procedures.

Learning Exercises

Complete the following review exercises after reading the associated pages in the textbook as indicated by each exercise. Answers to each review exercise are given at the end of the review exercises.

REVIEW EXERCISE A: Anatomy of Vascular System, Pulmonary and Systemic Circulation, and Cerebral Arteries and Veins (see textbook pp. 690-696)

1. List the two major divisions or components of the circulatory system:

    A. _____   B. _____

2. List the body system or part supplied by the following four divisions of the circulatory system:

    A. Cardio _____   C. Pulmonary _____

    B. Vascular _____   D. Systemic _____

3. List the three functions of the cardiovascular system:

    A. _____

    B. _____

    C. _____

4. Identify the major components of the general cardiovascular circulation as labeled on Fig. 21-1:

    A. _____

    B. _____

    C. _____

    D. _____

    E. _____

    F. _____

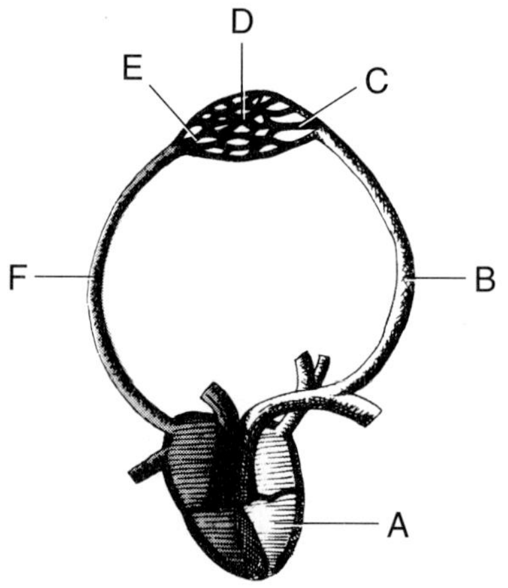

Fig. 21-1. Components of cardiovascular circulation.

5. Which of the six general components of the circulatory system, identified in question 4, carry oxygenated blood to

    body tissue? _____

6. Which of the six general components of the circulatory system carry deoxygenated blood?

    _____

7. For each of the following three blood components, list the function and the common term (unless no other term exists):

                    COMMON TERM   *FUNCTION*

    1. Erythrocytes   A. _____   B. _____

    2. Leukocytes   A. _____   B. _____

    3. Platelets   A. (no other term given)   B. _____

8. Plasma, the liquid portion of blood, consists of (A) _____% water and (B) _____% plasma protein and salts, nutrients, and oxygen.

9. Identify the chambers of the heart and the associated blood vessels (arteries and veins) as labeled on Fig. 21-2:

    A. _____ (chamber)

    B. _____ (chamber)

    C. _____ (chamber)

    D. _____

    E. _____

    F. _____

    G. _____

    H. _____

    I. _____

    J. _____ (chamber)

    K. _____

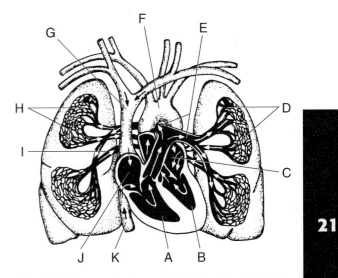

Fig. 21-2. Heart and pulmonary circulation (frontal view).

Questions 10 and 11 also relate to Fig. 21-2

10. In general, arteries carry oxygenated blood, and veins carry deoxygenated blood. The exceptions to these rules are:

    A. The _____ , which carry deoxygenated blood to the lungs

    B. The _____ , which carry oxygenated blood back to the atrium of the heart

11. A. Blood from the upper body returns to the heart through the _____ .

    B. Blood from the abdomen and the lower limbs returns through the _____ .

    C. Both of these major veins enter the _____ of the heart.

12. Identify the four major valves between the following heart chambers and associated vessels:

    A. Between right atrium and right ventricle: _____

    B. Between right ventricle and pulmonary arteries: _____

   C.   Between left atrium and left ventricle: _____

   D.   Between left ventricle and aorta: _____

13.   A.   The arteries that deliver blood to the heart muscle are the _____ .

   B.   These arteries originate at the _____ .

14.   List the three major branches of the coronary sinus:

   A.   _____   C.   _____

   B.   _____

15.   Identify the labeled arteries on this drawing (Fig. 21-3):

   A.   _____

   B.   _____

   C.   _____

   D.   _____

   E.   _____

   F.   _____

   G.   _____

   H.   _____

   I.   _____

   J.   _____

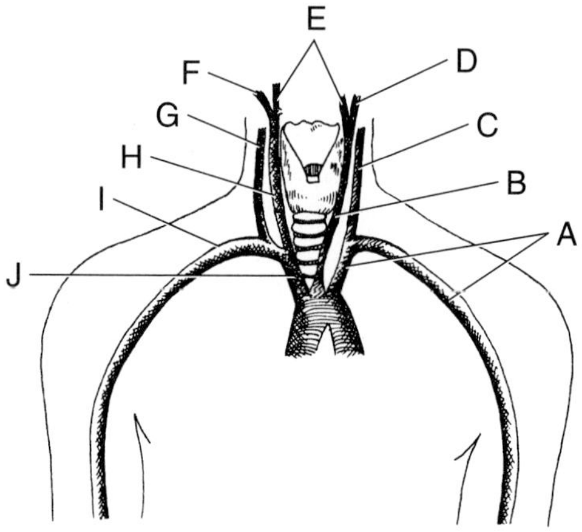

Fig. 21-3. Arterial branches of the aortic arch.

16.   List the three major branches of arteries arising from the arch of the aorta that supply the brain with blood:

   A.   _____   C.   _____

   B.   _____

17.   List the four major arteries supplying blood to the brain (important radiographically on a four-vessel angiogram).

   A.   _____   C.   _____

   B.   _____   D.   _____

18.   True/False: The brachiocephalic artery bifurcates to form the right common and right vertebral arteries.

19.   True/False: The level for bifurcation of the common carotid artery into the internal and external carotid arteries is at the level of C3-4.

20.   Any injection of the common carotid inferior to the bifurcation would result in filling both the

   _____ and _____ arteries.

21.   What is the name of the S-shaped portion of the internal carotid artery near the petrous portion of the temporal bone?

A.   Carotid sinus   C.   Carotid body

B.   Carotid canal   D.   Carotid siphon

22.   List the two end branches of the internal carotid artery:

A.   _____   B.   _____

23.   The _____ artery supplies much of the forebrain with blood.

24.   The _____ supply the posterior circulation of the brain.

25.   The two vertebral arteries unite to form the single _____ artery.

26.   Which of the two major branches of each internal carotid artery (**anterior cerebral** or **middle cerebral arteries**)

supply the lateral aspects of the cerebral hemispheres? _____

27.   The anterior and middle cerebral arteries superimpose one another to a greater extent on the

_____ (**lateral** or **frontal**) view.

28.   Identify which one of the four drawings below (Fig. 21-4) demonstrates each of the following:

1.   Middle cerebral artery and branches of the internal carotid artery _____

2.   Anterior cerebral artery and branches of the internal carotid artery _____

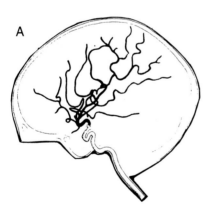

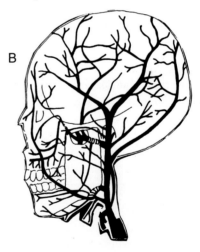

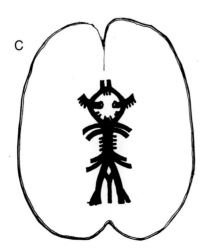

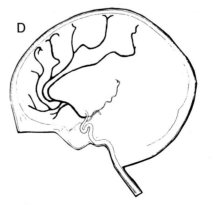

Fig. 21-4. Major cerebral arterial systems.

21

29. The posterior brain circulation communicates with the anterior circulation at the base of the brain in an arterial circle configuration called the circle of Willis (Fig. 21-5). Identify the five arteries or branches that make up the circle of Willis (labeled 1 through 5 on this drawing):

1. _____

2. _____

3. _____

4. _____

5. _____

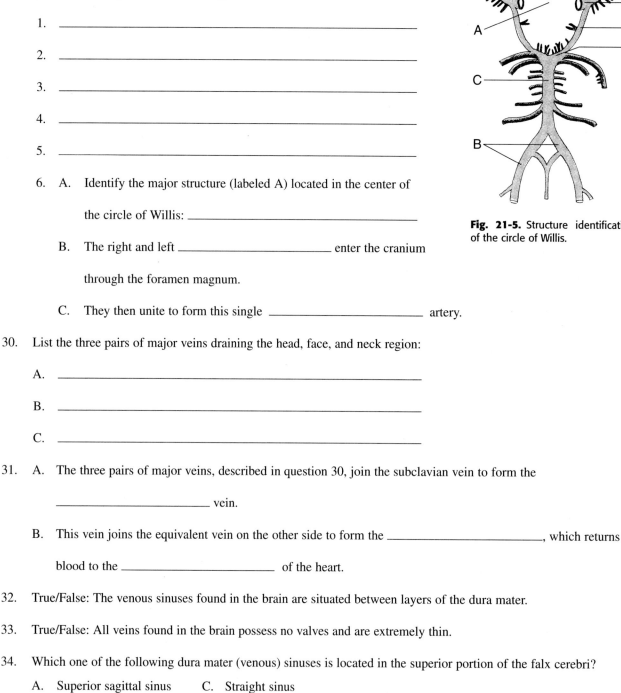

Fig. 21-5. Structure identification of the circle of Willis.

6. A. Identify the major structure (labeled A) located in the center of

      the circle of Willis: _____

   B. The right and left _____ enter the cranium

      through the foramen magnum.

   C. They then unite to form this single _____ artery.

30. List the three pairs of major veins draining the head, face, and neck region:

    A. _____

    B. _____

    C. _____

31. A. The three pairs of major veins, described in question 30, join the subclavian vein to form the

      _____ vein.

    B. This vein joins the equivalent vein on the other side to form the _____, which returns

      blood to the _____ of the heart.

32. True/False: The venous sinuses found in the brain are situated between layers of the dura mater.

33. True/False: All veins found in the brain possess no valves and are extremely thin.

34. Which one of the following dura mater (venous) sinuses is located in the superior portion of the falx cerebri?

    A. Superior sagittal sinus   C. Straight sinus

    B. Inferior sagittal sinus   D. Sigmoid sinus

35. Which bony landmark signifies the location of the confluence of venous sinuses?

    A. Foramen magnum   C. Internal occipital protuberance

    B. Petrous portion of temporal bone   D. Sella turcica

REVIEW EXERCISE B: Anatomy of Thoracic and Abdominal Arteries and Veins, Portal System, Upper and Lower Arteries and Veins, and Lymphatic System (see textbook pp. 697-701)

1. List the four segments of the thoracic section of the aorta as labeled on Fig. 21-6:

   A. _____

   B. _____

   C. _____

   D. _____

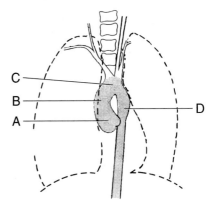

Fig. 21-6. Four segments of the aorta.

2. List the three common variations of the aortic arch that may be visualized during thoracic angiography and are demonstrated in Fig. 21-7:

   A. _____

   B. _____

   C. _____

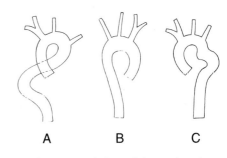

Fig. 21-7. Variations of the aortic arch.

3. Which one of the following veins receives blood from the intercostal, bronchial, esophageal, and phrenic veins?

   A. Pulmonary veins   B. Azygos vein   C. Inferior vena cava   D. Superior vena cava

4. List the five major branches of the abdominal aorta, labeled 1 through 5 on Fig. 21-8 (listed in order from most superior to most inferior):

   1. _____

   2. _____

   3. _____

   4. _____

   5. _____

5. List the three organs supplied with blood from the celiac artery, labeled A through C:

   A. _____

   B. _____

   C. _____

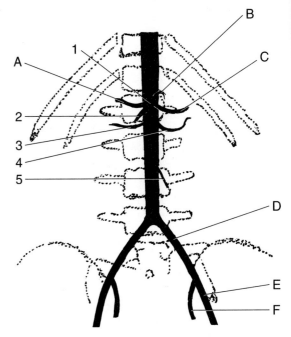

Fig. 21-8. Branches and divisions of the abdominal aorta.

21

List the divisions of the abdominal aorta as it enters the pelvic region, labeled D through F (Fig. 21-8):

D. _____

E. _____

F. _____

6. At what level does the descending aorta pass through the diaphragm to become the abdominal aorta?

A. T10   C. L1

B. T12   D. L2

7. The distal abdominal aorta bifurcates at the level of _____ vertebra.

8. Venous blood is returned to the heart from structures below the diaphragm through the inferior vena cava. Identify the major venous tributaries to the inferior vena cava, as labeled on Fig. 21-9:

A. _____

B. _____

C. _____

D. _____

E. Inferior vena cava

F. _____

G. _____

H. _____

I. _____

J. _____

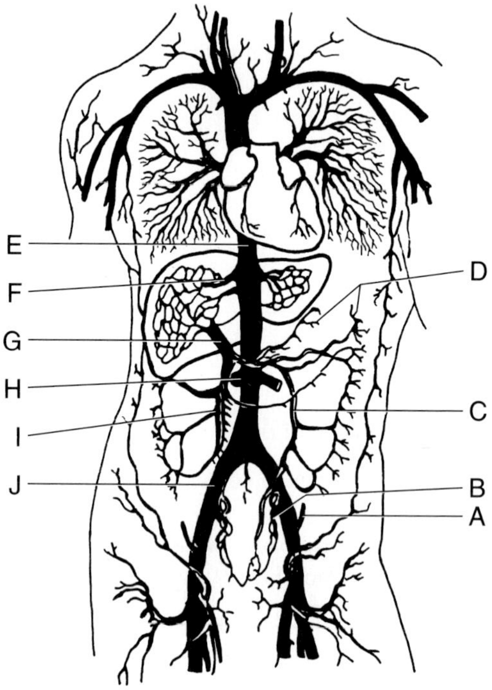

Fig. 21-9. Tributaries to the inferior vena cava.

9. Identify the following veins (A, B, D, and E) that make up the portal system, as labeled on Fig. 21-10. HINT: A and B are the two major veins that unite to form the hepatic portal vein (C).

A. _____

B. _____

C. Hepatic portal vein

D. _____ drain "filtered" blood from the

liver and return it to the:

E. _____

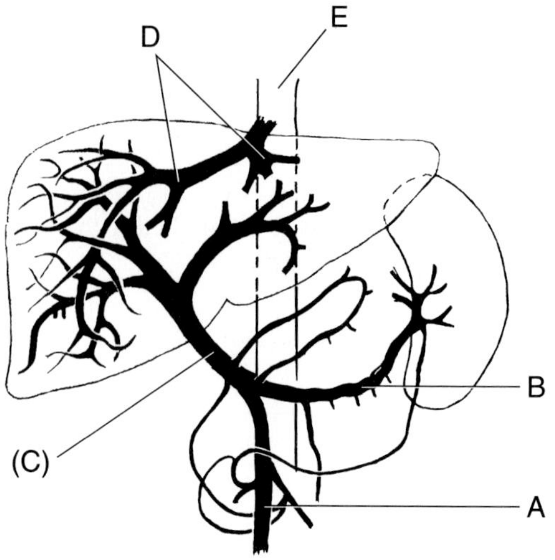

Fig. 21-10. Portal system.

10.   Identify the following upper limb arteries (Fig. 21-11):

On the right side of the body, (A) the _____ artery

gives rise to (B) the _____ artery.

Identify the following primary arteries of the upper limb, labeled *C* through *F*.

C.   _____

D.   _____

E.   _____

F.   _____

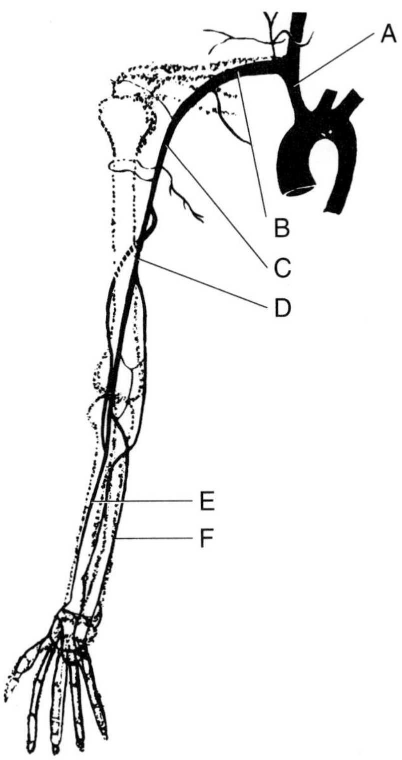

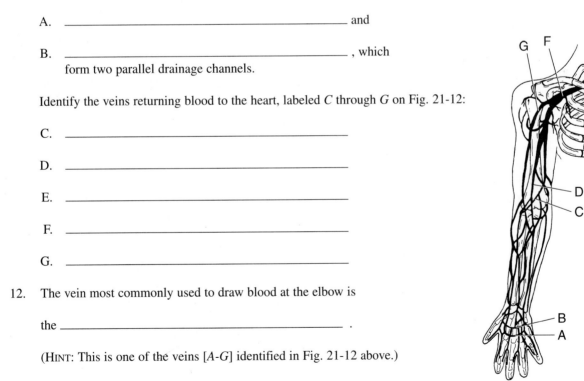

Fig. 21-11. Upper limb arteries.

11.   Identify the upper limb veins labeled on Fig. 21-12. The venous system of the upper and lower limbs may be divided into two sets. For the upper limb these begin with:

A.   _____ and

B.   _____ , which
form two parallel drainage channels.

Identify the veins returning blood to the heart, labeled *C* through *G* on Fig. 21-12:

C.   _____

D.   _____

E.   _____

F.   _____

G.   _____

12.   The vein most commonly used to draw blood at the elbow is

the _____ .

(HINT: This is one of the veins [*A-G*] identified in Fig. 21-12 above.)

Fig. 21-12. Upper limb veins.

Lower Limb Arteries (Fig. 21-13)

13.   Identify the following: The lower limb arterial system begins at the

   A.   _____ artery and continues as the

   B.   _____ artery until it divides into the

   C.   _____ and

   D.   _____ arteries in the area of the proximal and midfemur.

   At the knee this becomes the

   E.   _____ artery, which continues into the foot as the

   F.   _____ artery.

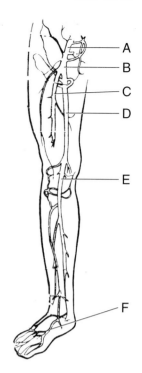

Fig. 21-13. Lower limb arteries.

Lower Limb Veins (Fig. 21-14)

14.   Identify the following labeled veins of the lower limb:

   A.   _____

   B.   _____

   C.   _____

   D.   _____

   E.   _____

   F.   _____

   G.   _____

   H.   _____

   I.   _____

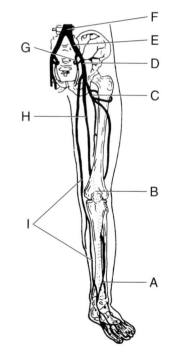

Fig. 21-14. Lower limb veins.

15.   The longest vein in the body is the _____ of the lower limb. (HINT: This is one of the labeled veins in Fig. 21-14.)

16.   Which duct in the lymphatic system receives interstitial fluid from the left side of the body, lower limbs, pelvis, and

   abdomen and drains this fluid into the left subclavian vein? _____ .

17. List the four functions of the lymphatic system:

A. _____

B. _____

C. _____

D. _____

18. True/False: Lymphatic fluid moves in two directions—toward and away from tissues.

19. The general term describing radiographic examination of the lymphatic **vessels and nodes** following injection of

contrast media is _____ .

20. Which imaging modality is replacing the procedure identified in question 19?

_____

21. True/False: There are thousands of lymph nodes in the body.

REVIEW EXERCISE C: Angiographic Procedures, Equipment, and Supplies (see textbook pp. 702-714)

1. Which of the following individuals is(are) not normally part of the angiographic team?
    A. Scrub nurse   C. Technologist
    B. Respiratory therapist   D. Radiologist

2. A common method or technique of introducing a needle and/or catheter into the blood vessel for angiographic

procedures is called the _____ .

3. In the correct order, list the six steps to the technique identified in question 2. Seldinger technique

A. _____   D. _____

B. _____   E. _____

C. _____   F. _____

4. In addition to the method listed above, what are two other techniques for accessing a vessel during angiography?

A. _____

B. _____

5. Which one of the following is not a common risk or complication of angiography?
    A. Embolus formation   C. Hypertension
    B. Dissection of a vessel D. Contrast media reaction

6. Which one of the following vessels is preferred for arterial vessel access for the majority of angiographic
    procedures?
    A. Femoral artery   C. Axillary artery
    B. Brachial artery   D. Common carotid artery

7. What is the primary purpose of premedicating the patient before an angiographic procedure?

    A. Reduce the risk for bleeding   C. Help the patient relax

    B. Reduce the risk for infection   D. All of the above

8. What type of contrast media is used for most angiographic procedures? _____

9. List the six most common complications associated with angiography:

    1. _____

    2. _____

    3. _____

    4. _____

    5. _____

    6. _____

10. List the three most common complications associated with a translumbar approach?

    1. _____

    2. _____

    3. _____

11. What is the minimum amount of time a patient should remain on bed rest following an invasive angiographic procedure?

    A. 1 hour   C. 4 hours

    B. 3 hours   D. 6 hours

12. At what degree angle should the head of the bed/stretcher be elevated following an invasive angiographic procedure?

    A. 10°   C. 20°

    B. 15°   D. 30°

13. True/False: Most pediatric angiographic procedures require patient sedation.

14. True/False: Angiographic rooms need to be considerably larger than conventional radiographic rooms.

15. Outlets for _____ and _____ should be located on the room walls

near the work area.

16. The two types of digital fluoroscopy and image acquisition systems include:

    A. _____

    B. _____

17. True/False: Flat detector angiographic systems require an image intensifier system.

18. True/False: The use of digital and/or digital subtraction angiography (DSA), as part of a PAC system, can eliminate the need for hard-copy images.

19. List three post processing options with digital imaging to improve or modify the image:

    A. _____

    B. _____

    C. _____

20. The purpose of the heating device on an electromechanical injector is

    _____ .

21. Flow rate for an automatic electromechanical injector is affected by viscosity of contrast media, injector pressure,

    and _____ and _____ of the catheter.

22. True/False: Computed tomography angiography (CTA) does not require the use of iodinated contrast media to demonstrate vascular structures.

23. True/False: Multislice CT can produce thinner slices and increase resolution of CTA images.

24. True/False: Magnetic resonance angiography (MRA) does not require the use of any type of contrast media or vessel puncture.

25. True/False: Rotational angiography units move around the anatomy up to 360° during the procedure.

26. True/False: Nuclear medicine complements other angiographic modalities even though it provides little anatomic detail.

27. True/False: Magnetic resonance angiography requires the use of special contrast media to demonstrate vasculature.

28. True/False: Color duplex ultrasound is effective in demonstrating thrombus formation in the circle of Willis in the adult.

29. True/False: Carbon dioxide is recommended instead of iodinated contrast media for carotid angiography.

30. True/False: Gadolinium is recommended for renal angiography for patients with known renal disease.

REVIEW EXERCISE D: Specific and Interventional Angiographic Procedures (see textbook pp. 715-721)

1. List the five common pathologic indicators for cerebral angiography.

   A. _____   D. _____

   B. _____   E. _____

   C. _____

2. The point of bifurcation is of special interest to the radiologist; at this point, the internal carotid artery is more

   _____ (**medial** or **lateral**) when compared with the external carotid on an AP projection.

3. List four vessels commonly demonstrated during cerebral angiography:

   A. _____

   B. _____

   C. _____

   D. _____

4. On an AP axial image taken during an internal carotid arteriogram, the floor of the anterior fossa and the

   _____ are superimposed.

5. List five specific pathologies that are common indications for thoracic and pulmonary angiography.

   A. _____

   B. _____

   C. _____

   D. _____

   E. _____

6. The most common pathologic indicator for **pulmonary** arteriography is _____ .

7. True/False: Pulmonary angiography is performed less often because of availability of alternative modalities such as high-resolution CT.

8. The preferred puncture site for a thoracic aortogram is the:

   A. Femoral vein   C. Pulmonary artery

   B. Pulmonary vein   D. Femoral artery

9. The preferred puncture site for a pulmonary arteriogram is:

   A. Femoral vein   C. Pulmonary artery

   B. Pulmonary vein   D. Femoral artery

10. What is the average amount of contrast media injected during a thoracic angiogram?

    A. 5 to 8 ml   C. 20 to 25 ml

    B. 10 to 15 ml   D. 30 to 50 ml

11. To prevent superimposition of the aortic arch with surrounding structures during a thoracic aortogram, a _____ °
    LAO is often performed.

    A. 5 to 10   C. 45

    B. 15 to 20   D. 60

12. Coronary angiography is typically a study of the:

    A. Coronary arteries   C. Coronary veins

    B. Aortic arch   D. Chambers of the heart

13. Which vessel is commonly catheterized for access to the right side of the heart? _____

14. The average imaging rate during angiocardiography is:

    A. 2 to 3 frames per second   C. 15 to 30 frames per second

    B. 8 to 10 frames per second   D. 45 to 60 frames per second

15. Which one of the following terms describes the pumping efficiency of the left ventricle?

    A. Ejection fraction   C. Ejection coefficient

    B. Systolic contraction ratio   D. Myocardial perfusion ratio

16. List five common pathologic indicators for abdominal angiography:

    A. _____

    B. _____

    C. _____

    D. _____

    E. _____

17. The common puncture site for selective abdominal angiography is the _____ artery using the Seldinger technique.

18. Superselective abdominal angiography can be performed to visualize specific branches (and associated organs) of the abdominal aorta. Which three branches are most commonly catheterized for this purpose?

    A. _____

    B. _____

    C. _____

19. The term for an angiographic study of the superior and inferior vena cava is _____ .

20. True/False: Venograms are rarely performed today because of increased use of color duplex ultrasound.

21. To study the left upper limb arteries, the catheter is passed from the aortic arch into the:

    A. Left common carotid   C. Left vertebral artery

    B. Left brachiocephalic vein   D. Left subclavian artery

22. True/False: Lymphography can be performed to diagnose Hodgkin's lymphoma.

23. Which one of the following conditions may contraindicate a lymphogram?

    A. Advanced pulmonary disease   C. Cervical cancer

    B. Prostate cancer   D. Peripheral swelling

24. What type of contrast agent is most often used for a lymphogram?

    A. Water-soluble iodinated-nonionic   C. Oil-based

    B. Water-soluble iodinated-ionic   D. Negative-CO_2

25. Why is a blue dye injected subcutaneously at the beginning of a lower limb lymphogram?

    A. Helps to identify lymph vessels   C. Anesthetizes lymph vessels

    B. Increases transit time of contrast media   D. Reduces risk for contrast media reaction

26. Indicate whether the following interventional procedures are vascular or nonvascular procedures:

    _____ 1. Percutaneous transluminal angioplasty (PTA)   A. Vascular procedure

    _____ 2. Infusion therapy   B. Nonvascular procedure

    _____ 3. Percutaneous biliary drainage (PBD)

    _____ 4. Percutaneous gastrostomy

    _____ 5. Stent placement

    _____ 6. Embolization

    _____ 7. Percutaneous abdominal drainage

    _____ 8. Nephrostomy

    _____ 9. Thrombolysis

    _____ 10. Percutaneous needle biopsy

    _____ 11. Kyphoplasty

    _____ 12. Transjugular intrahepatic portosystemic shunt (TIPS)

27. How is the hepatic portal system accessed during a TIPS procedure? _____

28. What vasoconstrictor is commonly given during infusion therapy to control bleeding? _____

29. What type of catheter is often used to retrieve urethral stones? _____

30. What is the name of the vertebroplasty technique performed to restore the collapsed portion of a vertebral body?

    _____

31. What specific device is placed within the collapsed vertebrae to restore its height and structure for the procedure

    identified in question 30? _____

32. What type of catheter is used for transluminal angioplasty? _____

33. What is the correct term describing the interventional procedure for dissolving a blood clot? _____

34. What drug is often coated on a drug-eluting stent to inhibit the regrowth of vascular tissue within a vessel?

    _____

35. Which one of the following pathologic indications is most common for performing a percutaneous biliary drainage (PBD)?

    A. Biliary obstruction   C. Posttraumatic biliary leakage

    B. Suppurative cholangitis   D. Unresectable malignant disease

36. True/False: Percutaneous abdominal drainage procedures have a success rate of only 50%.

37. True/False: Percutaneous gastrostomy is performed primarily for patients who are unable to eat orally.

38. True/False: Interventional angiographic procedures are used primarily for providing diagnostic information and secondarily for treatment of disease.

39. True/False: Interventional imaging procedures are most commonly performed in surgery.

40. Which of the following imaging modalities is recommended for biopsy of small, deep lesions surrounded by large vessels?

    A. Sonography   C. MRI

    B. CT   D. Digital fluoroscopy

21

Answers to Review Exercises

Review Exercise A: Anatomy of Cardiovascular System, Pulmonary and Systemic Circulation, and Cerebral Arteries and Veins

1. A. Cardiovascular
   B. Lymphatic
2. A. Heart
   B. Blood vessels
   C. Heart to lungs
   D. Throughout the body
3. A. Transportation of oxygen, nutrients, hormones, and chemicals
   B. Removal of waste products
   C. Maintenance of body temperature, water, and electrolyte balance
4. A. Heart
   B. Artery
   C. Arteriole
   D. Capillary
   E. Venule
   F. Vein
5. B (artery) and C (arteriole)
6. E (venule) and F (vein)
7. 1. A. Red blood cells
      B. Transports oxygen
   2. A. White blood cells
      B. Defends against infection and disease
   3. A. (no other term given)
      B. Repairs tears in blood vessels and promotes blood clotting
8. A. 92
   B. 7
9. A. Right ventricle
   B. Left ventricle
   C. Left atrium
   D. Capillaries of left lung
   E. Pulmonary arteries
   F. Aorta (arch)
   G. Superior vena cava
   H. Capillaries of right lung
   I. Pulmonary veins
   J. Right atrium
   K. Inferior vena cava
10. A. Pulmonary arteries
    B. Pulmonary veins
11. A. Superior vena cava
    B. Inferior vena cava
    C. Right atrium
12. A. Tricuspid valve
    B. Pulmonary (pulmonary semilunar) valve
    C. Mitral (bicuspid) valve
    D. Aortic (aortic semilunar) valve
13. A. Right and left coronary arteries
    B. Aortic bulb

14. A. Great cardiac vein
    B. Middle cardiac vein
    C. Small cardiac vein
15. A. Left subclavian
    B. Left common carotid
    C. Left vertebral
    D. Left internal carotid
    E. Right and left external carotids
    F. Right internal carotid
    G. Right vertebral
    H. Right common carotid
    I. Right subclavian
    J. Brachiocephalic
16. A. Brachiocephalic artery
    B. Left common carotid artery
    C. Left subclavian artery
17. A. Right common carotid artery
    B. Left common carotid artery
    C. Right vertebral artery
    D. Left vertebral artery
18. False (right common carotid and right subclavian)
19. True
20. Internal and external carotid
21. D. Carotid siphon
22. A. Anterior cerebral artery
    B. Middle cerebral artery
23. Anterior cerebral
24. Vertebrobasilar arteries
25. Basilar
26. Middle cerebral arteries
27. Lateral
28. 1. A
    2. D
29. 1. Posterior cerebral arteries
    2. Posterior communicating arteries
    3. Internal cerebral arteries
    4. Anterior cerebral arteries
    5. Anterior communicating artery
    6. A. Hypophysis (pituitary) gland
       B. Vertebral arteries
       C. Basilar
30. A. Right and left internal jugular veins
    B. Right and left external jugular veins
    C. Right and left vertebral veins
31. A. Brachiocephalic
    B. Superior vena cava; right atrium
32. True
33. True
34. A. Superior sagittal sinus
35. C. Internal occipital protuberance

Review Exercise B: Anatomy of Thoracic and Abdominal Arteries and Veins, Portal System, Upper and Lower Arteries and Veins, and Lymphatic System

1. A. Aortic bulb
   B. Ascending aorta
   C. Aortic arch
   D. Descending aorta
2. A. Left circumflex
   B. Inverse aorta
   C. Pseudocoarctation
3. B. Azygos vein
4. 1. Celiac axis artery
   2. Superior mesenteric artery
   3. Right renal artery
   4. Left renal artery
   5. Inferior mesenteric artery
5. A. Liver
   B. Spleen
   C. Stomach
   D. Left common iliac artery
   E. Left external iliac artery
   F. Left internal iliac artery
6. B. T12
7. L4
8. A. Left external iliac vein
   B. Left internal iliac vein
   C. Inferior mesenteric vein
   D. Splenic vein
   E. (Inferior vena cava)
   F. Hepatic vein
   G. Portal vein
   H. Right renal vein
   I. Superior mesenteric vein
   J. Right common iliac vein
9. A. Superior mesenteric vein
   B. Splenic vein
   C. (Hepatic portal vein)
   D. Hepatic veins
   E. Inferior vena cava
10. A. Brachiocephalic
    B. Subclavian
    C. Axillary
    D. Brachial
    E. Radial
    F. Ulnar
11. A. Superficial palmar arch vein
    B. Deep palmar arch vein
    C. Median cubital
    D. Brachial
    E. Superior vena cava
    F. Subclavian
    G. Cephalic
12. Median cubital vein
13. A. External iliac
    B. Common femoral
    C. Deep femoral

21

D. Femoral
E. Popliteal
F. Dorsalis pedis
14. A. Anterior tibial
B. Popliteal
C. Deep femoral
D. External iliac
E. Left common iliac
F. Inferior vena cava
G. Internal iliac
H. Femoral
I. Great saphenous
15. Great saphenous vein
16. Thoracic duct
17. A. Fights diseases by producing lymphocytes and microphages
B. Returns proteins and other substances to the blood
C. Filters lymph in the lymph nodes
D. Transfers fats from the intestine to the blood
18. False (one direction—away from tissues)
19. Lymphography
20. Computed tomography
21. True

Review Exercise C: Angiographic Procedures, Equipment, and Supplies

1. B. Respiratory therapist
2. Seldinger technique
3. A. Insertion of needle
B. Placement of needle in lumen of vessel
C. Insertion of guide wire
D. Removal of needle
E. Threading of catheter to area of interest
F. Removal of guide wire
4. A. Cutdown
B. Translumbar approach
5. C. Hypertension
6. A. Femoral artery
7. C. Help the patient relax
8. Water-soluble, nonionic contrast media
9. 1. Bleeding at the puncture site
2. Thrombus formation
3. Embolus formation
4. Dissection of a vessel
5. Infection of puncture site
6. Contrast media reaction

10. 1. Hemothorax
2. Pneumothorax
3. Retroperitoneal hemorrhage
11. C. 4 hours
12. D. 30°
13. True
14. True
15. Oxygen and suction
16. A. Analog-to-digital conversion
B. Flat detector—direct digital conversion
17. False
18. True
19. A. Pixel-shifting or remasking
B. Magnified or zooming
C. Quantitative analysis of image to measure distances and calculate stenosis
20. To maintain temperature of contrast media at body temperature
21. Length and diameter
22. False (does require contrast media)
23. True
24. True
25. False (only 180°)
26. True
27. False (does not require contrast media)
28. False
29. False
30. False

Review Exercise D: Specific and Interventional Angiographic Procedures

1. A. Vascular stenosis and occlusions
B. Aneurysms
C. Trauma
D. Arteriovenous malformations
E. Neoplastic disease
2. Lateral
3. A. Common carotid arteries
B. Internal carotid arteries
C. External carotid arteries
D. Vertebral arteries
4. Petrous ridges
5. A. Aneurysm
B. Congenital abnormalities
C. Vessel stenosis
D. Embolus
E. Trauma
6. Pulmonary embolus
7. True

8. D. Femoral artery
9. A. Femoral vein
10. D. 30 to 50 ml
11. C. 45
12. A. Coronary arteries
13. Femoral vein
14. C. 15 to 30 frames per second
15. A. Ejection fraction
16. A. Aneurysm
B. Congenital abnormality
C. GI bleed
D. Stenosis or occlusion
E. Trauma
17. Femoral
18. A. Renal arteries
B. Celiac artery
C. Superior and inferior mesenteric arteries
19. Venacavography
20. True
21. D. Left subclavian artery
22. True
23. A. Advanced pulmonary disease
24. C. Oil-based
25. A. Helps to identify lymph vessels
26. 1. A
2. A
3. B
4. B
5. A
6. A
7. B
8. B
9. A
10. B
11. B
12. A
27. Through the right jugular vein
28. Vasopressin (Pitressin)
29. Basket catheter or loop snare
30. Kyphoplasty
31. Kyphoplasty balloon
32. Balloon catheter
33. Thrombolysis
34. Taxol®
35. D. Unresectable malignant disease
36. False (70% to 80%)
37. True
38. False (primarily for treatment of disease)
39. False (performed primarily in angiographic suite)
40. B. CT

SELF-TEST

My Score = _____ %

Directions: This self-test should be taken only after completing all of the readings, review exercises, and laboratory activities for a particular section. The purpose of this test is not only to provide a good learning exercise but also to serve as a good indicator of what your final evaluation exam will be. It is strongly suggested that if you do not get at least a 90% to 95% grade on this self-test, you review those areas in which you missed questions before going to your instructor for the final evaluation exam for this chapter. (There are 80 questions or blanks—each is worth 1.25 points.)

1. The two arteries that deliver blood to the heart muscle are:

    A. Right and left pulmonary veins   C. Right and left pulmonary arteries

    B. Right and left brachiocephalic arteries   D. Right and left coronary arteries

2. Which of the following arteries does not originate directly from the arch of the aorta?

    A. Brachiocephalic   C. Left common carotid

    B. Left subclavian   D. Right common carotid

3. Each common carotid artery bifurcates into the internal and external arteries at the level of:

    A. C4 vertebra   C. C2 vertebra

    B. C6 vertebra   D. C2 vertebra

4. Which vessels carry oxygenated blood from the lungs back to the heart?

    A. Pulmonary veins   C. Coronary arteries

    B. Pulmonary arteries   D. Aorta

5. Which of the following arteries arises from the brachiocephalic artery rather than the aortic arch?

    A. Right vertebral   C. Right common carotid

    B. Left vertebral   D. Left common carotid

6. The external carotid does not supply blood to the:

    A. Anterior portion of brain   C. Anterior neck

    B. Facial area   D. Greater part of the scalp and meninges

7. Two branches of each internal carotid artery, which are well visualized with an internal carotid arteriogram, are the:

    A. Posterior and middle cerebral arteries   C. Right and left vertebral arteries

    B. Anterior and middle cerebral arteries   D. Facial and maxillary arteries

8. The two vertebral arteries enter the cranium through the foramen magnum and unite to form the:

    A. Brachiocephalic artery   C. Circle of Willis

    B. Vertebrobasilar artery   D. Basilar artery

9. The basilar artery rests upon the clivus of the _____ bone.

    A. Ethmoid   C. Temporal

    B. Parietal   D. Sphenoid

10. Which of the following veins do not drain blood from the head, face, and neck regions?

   A. Right and left internal jugular veins   C. Internal and external cerebral veins

   B. Right and left vertebral veins   D. Right and left external jugular veins

11. The superior and inferior sagittal sinuses join certain other sinuses, such as the transverse sinus, at the base of the brain to become the:

   A. External jugular vein   C. Subclavian vein

   B. Internal jugular vein   D. Vertebral vein

12. Which vein receives blood from the intercostal, esophageal, and phrenic veins?

   A. Superior vena cava   C. Azygos vein

   B. Inferior vena cava   D. Brachiocephalic vein

13. Match the following abdominal arteries with the labeled parts on Fig. 21-15:

   _____   1. Inferior mesenteric

   _____   2. Superior mesenteric

   _____   3. Left renal

   _____   4. Right renal

   _____   5. Common hepatic

   _____   6. Celiac (trunk) axis

   _____   7. Left common iliac

   _____   8. Left internal iliac

   _____   9. Left external iliac

   _____   10. Left gastric

   _____   11. Abdominal aorta

   _____   12. Splenic

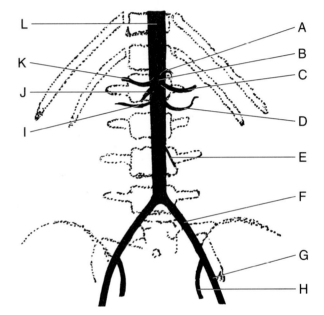

Fig. 21-15. Abdominal arteries.

14. True/False: The right subclavian artery arises directly from the aortic arch.

15. True/False: The cephalic vein is most commonly used for venipuncture.

16. True/False: The great saphenous vein is the longest vein in the body.

17. True/False: The thoracic duct is the largest lymph vessel in the body.

18. What is another term for the aortic bulb?

   A. Aortic stem   C. Aortic root

   B. Aortic confluence   D. Aortic sphincter

19. How many segments make up the thoracic aorta?

    A. Three   C. Five

    B. Four   D. Two

20. A condition in which the aortic arch is located in the right side of the thorax is a variation termed:

    A. Left circumflex aorta   C. Pseudocoarctation

    B. Inverse aorta   D. Situs inversus

21. Which of the following vessels carries blood from the intestine to the liver for filtration?

    A. Portal vein   C. Superior mesenteric vein

    B. Hepatic veins   D. Inferior vena cava

22. Which one of the following functions is *not* performed by the lymphatic system?

    A. Produce lymphocytes and microphages   C. Filter the lymph

    B. Synthesize simple carbohydrates   D. Return proteins and other substances to the blood

23. Solid food should be withheld for approximately _____ hours before an angiographic procedure.

    A. 1   C. 8

    B. 4   D. 24

24. Which of the following vessels is most often punctured for the Seldinger technique?

    A. Abdominal aorta   C. Femoral artery

    B. Femoral vein   D. Axillary artery

21

25.   Match each of the following terms with its definition or description:

_____   1.   Also known as *red blood cells*

_____   2.   Component of blood that helps repair tears in
            blood vessel walls and promotes blood clotting

_____   3.   Carries deoxygenated blood from the right
            ventricle of the heart to the lungs

_____   4.   Heart valve found between the left atrium and
            left ventricle

_____   5.   Heart valve found between the right atrium and
            right ventricle

_____   6.   The vessels that provide blood to the heart muscle

_____   7.   The artery that bifurcates to form the right
            common carotid and right subclavian artery

_____   8.   The artery that primarily supplies blood to the
            anterior neck, scalp, and meninges

_____   9.   The artery that bifurcates into the anterior and
            middle cerebral artery

_____   10.   The aspect of the sphenoid bone upon which the
            basilar artery rests

_____   11.   The membranous portion of the dura mater
            containing the superior sagittal sinus

_____   12.   The artery that forms the left gastric, hepatic,
            and splenic arteries

_____   13.   The vein created by the splenic and superior
            mesenteric veins

_____   14.   The vessel that carries oxygenated blood from
            the lungs to the left atrium of the heart

_____   15.   A radiographic study of the lymph vessels

A.   Brachiocephalic artery

B.   Pulmonary veins

C.   Celiac artery

D.   Coronary arteries

E.   Superior vena cava

F.   Portal vein

G.   Falx cerebri

H.   Lymphangiogram

I.   Inferior mesenteric artery

J.   Coronary sinu

K.   External carotid artery

L.   Tricuspid valve

M.   Clivus

N.   Mitral (bicuspid) valve

O.   Erythrocytes

P.   Pulmonary artery

Q.   Platelets

R.   Internal carotid artery

26.   Injection flow rate in angiography is *not* affected by:

A.   Viscosity of contrast media   C.   Body temperature

B.   Length and diameter of catheter   D.   Injection pressure

27.   Which one of the following imaging modalities will best demonstrate velocity of blood flow within a vessel?

A.   Computed tomography angiography   C.   Magnetic resonance imaging

B.   Color duplex ultrasound   D. CO_2 angiography

28. What is the minimum amount of time a patient should remain on bed rest following an angiographic procedure?

    A. 1 hour   C. 8 hours

    B. 4 hours   D. 24 hours

29. What type of angiographic imaging system does not require the use of image intensifier or video camera?

    A. C-arm conventional fluoroscopy   C. Pulsed generator fluoroscopy

    B. Analog-to-digital conversion fluoroscopy   D. Flat detector fluoroscopy

30. True/False: Cut film changers are still commonly used for angiography.

31. True/False: Multislice CT scanning does not require arterial puncture and catheter insertion to demonstrate vascular structures.

32. True/False: Contrast media must be used during magnetic resonance angiography.

33. True/False: CO_2 angiography requires the use of a special injector.

34. Which of the following is *not* a pathologic indicator for cerebral angiography?

    A. Vascular lesions   C. Coarctation

    B. Aneurysm   D. Arteriovenous malformation

35. The imaging sequence during cerebral angiography typically requires _____ to include all phases of circulation (arterial to venous).

    A. 1 to 3 seconds   C. 8 to 10 seconds

    B. 4 to 6 seconds   D. 12 to 15 seconds

36. Pulmonary arteriography is most often performed to diagnose:

    A. Heart valve disease   C. Arteriovenous malformation

    B. Pulmonary emboli   D. Coarctation of the aorta

37. The most common vascular approach during pulmonary arteriography is the:

    A. Femoral vein   C. Superior vena cava

    B. Femoral artery   D. Axillary artery

38. Which one of the following positions will prevent superimposition of the proximal aorta and aortic arch during a thoracic aortogram?

    A. 45° RPO   C. 45° LAO

    B. 45° LPO   D. Lateral

39. During angiocardiography, the catheter is advanced from the aorta into the:

    A. Superior vena cava   C. Left ventricle

    B. Right ventricle   D. Brachiocephalic artery

40. The imaging rate during angiocardiography is between:

    A. 1 to 3 frames per second   C. 10 to 12 frames per second

    B. 4 to 8 frames per second   D. 15 to 30 frames per second

21

41. Which of the following would not be a common pathologic indicator for abdominal angiography?

    A. Aneurysm   C. Trauma

    B. Stenosis or occlusions of aorta   D. Bowel obstruction

42. The average amount of contrast media injected during a venacavogram is:

    A. 6 to 8 ml   C. 30 to 40 ml

    B. 10 to 15 ml   D. 50 to 70 ml

43. True/False: Venograms of the extremity are rarely performed today because of the increased sensitivity of color duplex ultrasound.

44. Why is a blue dye injected during a lymphogram?

    A. Helps to visualize the lymph vessels   C. Helps to identify the veins of the limb

    B. Anesthetizes the vessels   D. Reduces spasm of the lymph vessels

45. True/False: Images are often taken 24 hours following injection during a lymphogram.

46. True/False: The most common contrast agent used during lymphography is water-soluble and nonionic.

47. The most common pathologic indication for chemoembolization is to treat:

    A. Brain aneurysm   C. AV malformation

    B. Stenosed vessels   D. Malignancies

48. Match the following descriptions to the correct term or interventional procedure (use each choice only once).

    _____ A. Intravascular administration of drugs   1. Embolization

    _____ B. Device to extract urethral stones   2. Nephrostomy

    _____ C. Procedure to dissolve blood clots   3. Infusion therapy

    _____ D. Technique to restrict uncontrolled hemorrhage   4. Basket or loop snare catheter

    _____ E. Technique to decompress obstructed bile duct   5. Percutaneous gastrostomy

    _____ F. Direct puncture and catheterization of the renal pelvis   6. Thrombolysis

    _____ G. Placement of an extended feeding tube into the stomach   7. Percutaneous biliary drainage

49. True/False: A vena cava filter is placed superior to the renal veins to prevent renal vein thrombosis.

50. True/False: The TIPS procedure involves placement of an intrahepatic stent.

CHAPTER 22

Computed Tomography

This chapter presents the general principles of computed tomography (CT) and the various equipment systems in use today. A study of soft tissue anatomy of the central nervous system (CNS) as viewed in axial sections is included. An introduction into the purpose, pathologic indications, and procedure of cranial, thoracic, abdominal, and pelvic computed tomography is also covered in this chapter. Selected sectional images of these three regions are presented.

CHAPTER OBJECTIVES

After you have successfully completed the activities of this chapter, you will be able to:

_____ 1. List the two general divisions of the CNS.

_____ 2. Identify the specialized cells (neurons) of the nervous system and describe their specific parts and functions.

_____ 3. List the specific membranes or coverings of the CNS and identify the meningeal spaces or potential spaces associated with them.

_____ 4. List the three primary divisions of the brain.

_____ 5. List the four major cavities of the ventricular system and identify specific structures and passageways of the ventricular system.

_____ 6. Identify select gray and white matter structures in the brain.

_____ 7. Describe the concept of the "blood-brain barrier."

_____ 8. List the twelve cranial nerves.

_____ 9. List three advantages of computed tomography over conventional radiography.

_____ 10. Identify the generational changes and advances in computed tomography (CT) systems.

_____ 11. List the major components of a computed tomographic (CT) system.

_____ 12. Explain the basic operating principles of computed tomography imaging, including x-ray transmission, data acquisition, image reconstruction, window width, window level, and slice thickness.

_____ 13. Define and calculate the pitch ratio for a helical CT scan using different variables.

_____ 14. Identify the scan parameters for cranial, thoracic, abdominal, and pelvic computed tomography studies.

_____ 15. Identify specific structures of the brain, thorax, abdomen, and pelvis seen on axial drawings and CT sectional images.

Learning Exercises

The following review exercises should be completed only after careful study of the associated pages in the textbook as indicated by each exercise. Answers to each review exercise are given at the end of the review exercises.

REVIEW EXERCISE A: Anatomy of the Central Nervous System (see textbook pp. 724-732)

1. The central nervous system can be divided into the following two main divisions:

    A. _____

    B. _____

2. A. The solid spinal cord terminates at the level of the lower border of which vertebra? _____

    B. This tapered terminal area of the spinal cord is called the _____ .

3. A. The specialized cells of the nervous system that conduct electrical impulses are called _____ .

    B. The parts of these cells that receive the electrical impulse and conduct them *toward* the cell body are called

    _____ .

4. Three membranes or layers of coverings called *meninges* enclose both the brain and the spinal cord. Certain important spaces or potential spaces are associated with these meninges. List these three meninges and three associated spaces as described below:

MENINGES	*SPACES*
Skull or cranium	
A. _____	D. _____
(Outer "hard" or "tough" layer)	(Space or potential space)
B. _____	E. _____
(Spiderlike avascular membrane)	(Narrow space containing thin layer of fluid)
C. _____	F. _____
(Inner "tender" layer)	(Wider space filled with cerebrospinal fluid)

5. The outer "hard" or "tough" membrane described above has an inner and outer layer tightly fused except for certain larger spaces between folds or creases of the brain and the skull, which provide for large venous blood channels

    called _____ .

6. The large cerebrum is divided into right and left hemispheres. Each hemisphere of the cerebrum is further divided into five lobes, with four of the lobes lying under the cranial bone of the same name. List these five lobes:

    A. _____   D. _____

    B. _____   E. _____

    C. _____

7. The brain (encephalon) can be divided into three general divisions: the (1) forebrain, (2) midbrain, and (3) hindbrain. The forebrain and hindbrain are both divided into three divisions. List the three divisions of the forebrain and the hindbrain as labeled on Fig. 22-1. (NOTE: Secondary terms for these divisions as found in the textbook are included in parentheses.)

    1. Forebrain   A. _____

        (Prosencephalon)   (Telencephalon)—Largest division

        (Diencephalon)   B. _____

                               C. _____

    2. Midbrain

        (Mesencephalon)

    3. Hindbrain   D. _____

        (Rhombencephalon)   E. _____

                               F. _____

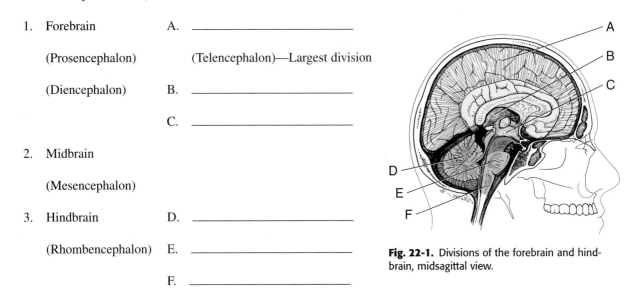

Fig. 22-1. Divisions of the forebrain and hindbrain, midsagittal view.

8. Identify the three lobes of the right cerebral hemisphere as labeled *A* through *C* in Fig. 22-2. The deep fissure separating the two cerebral hemispheres is labeled *D*. (NOTE: There is a fold of dura mater, called the *falx cerebri*, that extends deep within this fissure, separating the two hemispheres that is visualized on CT scans.)

    A. _____ lobe

    B. _____ lobe

    C. _____ lobe

    D. _____ fissure

9. The surface of each cerebral hemisphere contains numerous grooves and convolutions or raised areas. Identify labeled parts *E* through *G* in Fig. 22-2. Two of these raised areas, *E* and *G*, have specific names and are frequently demonstrated and identified on cranial CT scans. Part *F* is a shallow groove with a specific name.

    E. _____

    F. _____

    G. _____

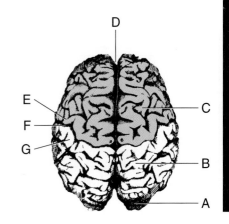

Fig. 22-2. Structures of the cerebral hemispheres.

22

10. What is the name of the arched mass of transverse fibers (white matter) that connects the two cerebral hemispheres?

    A. Falx cerebri   C. Central sulcus

    B. Anterior central gyrus D. Corpus callosum

11. What is the name of the large groove that separates the cerebral hemispheres?

    A. Anterior central gyrus C. Central sulcus

    B. Longitudinal fissure   D. Posterior central gyrus

12. The fluid manufactured and stored in the ventricular system is called (A) _____ ,

    abbreviated as (B) _____ . This fluid completely surrounds the brain and spinal

    cord by filling the space called the (C) _____ space. A blockage within this system may

    result in excessive accumulation of this fluid within the ventricles, creating a condition known as (D)

    _____ .

13. The cerebrospinal fluid–filled space and ventricular system are important in computed tomography because these areas can be differentiated from tissue structures by their density differences.

    A. The larger spaces or areas within the CSF-filled space are called _____ .

    B. The largest of these is the _____ , located just posterior and inferior to the fourth

       ventricle.

14. The central midline portion of the brain connecting the midbrain, pons, and medulla to the spinal cord is called the

    _____ .

15. A. The optic chiasma, the site where some of the optic nerves cross to the opposite side, is located in the

       _____ , a division of the forebrain.

    B. An important gland, which is located just inferior to this division of the forebrain, is the

       _____ .

16. A second important midline structure gland is the (A) _____ , which is located just superior

    to the (B) _____ , a division of the hindbrain.

17. The CNS can be divided by appearance into white matter and gray matter, which can be differentiated by CT. The difference in appearance between these two results from their makeup. Describe this difference by indicating what each consists of:

    A. White matter: _____

    B. Gray matter: _____

18. In general, the thin, outer cerebral cortex is (A) _____ matter, whereas the more centrally

    located brain tissue is (B) _____ matter.

19. List the three significant structures associated with the hypothalamus:

A. _____   B. _____   C. _____

20. List the three primary structures of the brain stem:

A. _____   B. _____   C. _____

21. Which aspect of the brain serves as an interpretation center for certain sensory impulses?

A. Midbrain   C. Thalamus

B. Pituitary gland   D. Hypothalamus

22. Which aspect of the brain coordinates important motor functions such as coordination, posture, and balance?

A. Pons   C. Midbrain

B. Cerebellum   D. Cerebrum

23. Which aspect of the brain controls important body activities related to homeostasis?

A. Pons   C. Thalamus

B. Cerebellum   D. Hypothalamus

24. Which structure of the brain controls a wide range of body functions, including growth and reproductive functions?

A. Pineal gland   C. Thalamus

B. Pituitary gland   D. Hypothalamus

25. List the four groupings of cerebral nuclei (basal ganglia):

A. _____   C. _____

B. _____   D. _____

26. Ventricles: There are four cavities in the ventricular system. These are labeled in Fig. 22-3 and demonstrate the four ventricles in relationship to other brain structures. Two of the ventricles are located within the right and left cerebral hemispheres (*A*); the remaining two are midline structures (*B* and *C*).

    The larger two ventricles (*A*) have four significant parts labeled *1, 2, 3,* and *6* in Fig. 22-4. The small ductlike structure (*4*) provides communication between ventricles, and number *5* indicates a connection between the third and fourth ventricles. An important gland (*8*) is also shown. Number *7* represents an important communication with the subarachnoid space on each side of the fourth ventricle.

    Identify the ventricles and their parts as labeled on these two drawings:

Fig. 22-3

A. Right and left _____ ventricles

B. _____ ventricle

C. _____ ventricle

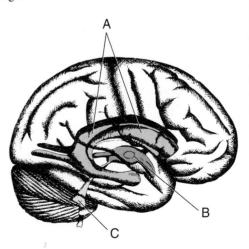

Fig. 22-3. Cavities in the ventricular system.

Fig. 22-4

1. _____ (occipital)

2. _____

3. _____ (frontal)

4. _____ (foramen)

5. _____

6. _____ (temporal)

7. _____

8. _____ (gland)

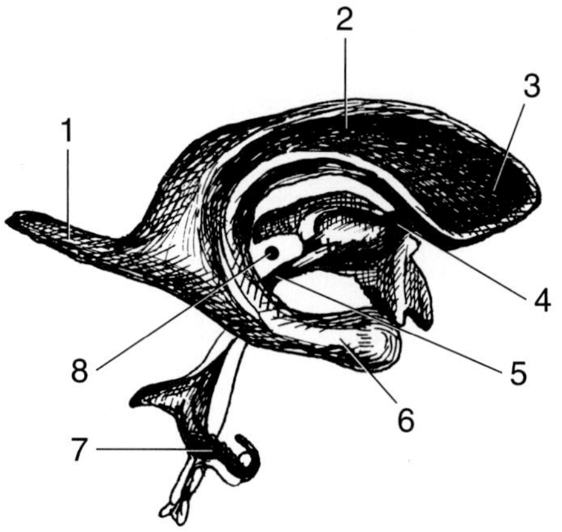

Fig. 22-4. Anatomy of the ventricles.

27. There are 12 pairs of cranial nerves, most of which originate from the brainstem and travel to various parts of the brain, controlling both sensory and motor functions. List these 12 pairs of cranial nerves:

A. _____   E. _____   I. _____

B. _____   F. _____   J. _____

C. _____   G. _____   K. _____

D. _____   H. _____   L. _____

REVIEW EXERCISE B: Basic Principles of Computed Tomography (CT) (see textbook pp. 733-737)

1. List the four advantages of CT over conventional radiography:

A. _____

B. _____

C. _____

D. _____

2. Match the following characteristics with the correct generation of CT scanner (answers may be used more than once, and some blanks have more than one answer):

   _____ 1. First scanner with fan-shaped beam and 30 or more detectors   A. First-generation

   _____ 2. 1- to 2-detector system   B. Second-generation

   _____ 3. 8 times faster than a 1-second, single-slice scanner   C. Third-generation

   _____ 4. First scanner to rotate a full 360° around patient   D. Fourth-generation

   _____ 5. Capable of volume scanning (multiple answers)   E. Multislice scanner

   _____ 6. 1 minute scan time for entire exam (multiple answers)

   _____ 7. Contains a bank of up to 960 detectors

   _____ 8. Scan times of 4½ minutes per slice

   _____ 9. 4800 or more detectors on a fixed ring

   _____ 10. Continuous volume scanning (CVS) (multiple answers)

   _____ 11. The first type with fixed detectors rather than detectors rotating with x-ray tube

   _____ 12. Capable of acquiring four or more slices simultaneously

   _____ 13. First scanner with larger aperture, which permitted full body scanning

3. True/False: The primary difference between each generation of CT scanners was the speed of the system.

4. True/False: Noninvasive studies of the heart are possible with multislice CT.

5. True/False: Volume CT scanners are limited to one 360° rotation per slice in the same direction.

6. True/False: Volume CT scanners are classified as either third- or fourth-generation scanners.

7. Which of the following devices replaced high-tension cables in helical CT scanners?

   A. Microswitches   C. Slip rings

   B. Variable diodes   D. Optic fiber lines

8. Which of the following is *not* an advantage of multislice CT scanners?

   A. Fast imaging speed   C. Minimizes patient motion

   B. Acquires large number of slices rapidly   D. Low-cost system to operate

9. The actual thickness of tomographic slices with multislice CT systems can range from:

   A. 1 to 3 or 4 centimeters   C. ¼ to 1 or more centimeters

   B. 0.5 millimeters or higher   D. 10 to 40 or more millimeters

10. List the three primary components of a computed tomographic system:

   A. _____   C. _____

   B. _____

22

11. Which part of the CT system houses the x-ray tube, detector array, and collimators? _____

12. The central opening in the CT support structure where the patient is scanned is called the _____ .

13. List the scintillation materials that make up the solid-state detector array: _____

14. The actual thickness of a tomographic slice is determined by:

    A. Detectors   C. Effective focal spot

    B. Prepatient collimator   D. Postpatient collimator

15. With a 512- × 512-image matrix, the CT computer must perform _____ mathematical calculations per slice.

    A. 128   C. 187,818

    B. 1280   D. 262,144

16. Image archiving for most modern CT systems is performed through a(n):

    A. PACS   C. Optical disk

    B. Magnetic disk or tape   D. Laser printer

17. What do the detectors measure in a CT system? _____

18. What is the meaning of the term *voxel*? _____

19. A voxel is a _____ dimensional image of the tissue, whereas a pixel represents only _____ dimensions.

20. The depth of the voxels is determined by:

    A. Slice thickness   C. Actual scan time

    B. Speed of computer   D. Size of the pixel

21. Data sets from image voxels are called:

    A. Bytes   C. Dimensions

    B. Isotropic   D. Spatial differences

22. Pixels represent varying degrees of:

    A. Resolution   C. Attenuation

    B. Contrast   D. Scatter radiation

23. Air would have a _____ (**higher** or **lower**) differential absorption as compared with soft tissue.

24. CT numbers are a numerical scale that represent tissue _____ .

25. List the general CT number or range for the following tissue types:

    A. Cortical bone _____

    B. White brain matter _____

    C. Blood _____

    D. Fat _____

    E. Lung tissue _____

    F. Air _____

    G. Water _____

26. Which medium serves as the baseline for CT numbers? _____

27. Match the most common appearance of the following tissue types as displayed on a CT image:

    _____ A. Bone   1. White

    _____ B. Gray brain matter   2. Gray

    _____ C. CSF   3. Black

    _____ D. Iodinated contrast media

28. **Window width** (WW) controls:

    A. Displayed image density   C. Slice thickness
    B. Displayed image contrast   D. Total number of slices

29. **Window level** (WL) controls:

    A. Image brightness   C. Slice thickness
    B. Image contrast   D. Total number of slices

30. Pitch is defined as:

    _____

31. Pitch is a relationship between _____ and _____ .

32. Calculate the pitch ratio using the following parameters: Couch movement at a rate of 20 mm per second with a

    slice collimation of 10 mm _____ .

33. The pitch ratio calculated in question 32 is an example of:

    A. Undersampling   C. Perfect pitch
    B. Oversampling   D. Intermittent pitch

22

34. Which of the following parameters would produce a 0.5:1.0 pitch ratio?

A. 10-mm couch movement and 10-mm slice thickness

B. 15-mm couch movement and 10-mm slice thickness

C. 10-mm couch movement and 20-mm slice thickness

D. 30-mm couch movement and 10-mm slice thickness

REVIEW EXERCISE C: Clinical Applications of Head CT and Sectional Anatomy of the Brain
(see textbook pp. 738-742)

1. A scanogram or topogram is another term for:

A. CT scan of the head   C. Warm up procedure for scanner

B. Scout view   D. Calibration procedure for scanner

2. Approximately _____% to _____% of all cranial CTs require contrast media.

3. True/False: Oxygen deprivation of **2 minutes** will lead to permanent brain cell injury.

4. True/False: Iodinated contrast media is able to pass through the blood brain barrier in the normal individual.

5. True/False: Iodinated contrast media are often required to visualize neoplasms during a head CT scan.

6. Which one of the following substances will not pass through the blood-brain barrier?

A. Proteins   C. Oxygen

B. Glucose   D. Select ions found in the blood

7. True/False: Patient dose is higher for a CT scan of the head as compared with a routine skull series.

8. True/False: The higher the pitch ratio during a helical scan, the greater the patient dose.

9. Head CT images are viewed in what two window settings?

A. _____

B. _____

10. The most important aspect of positioning the head for cranial CT is to ensure there is no

_____ and no _____ of the head.

11. Trauma to the skull may lead to a collection of blood accumulating under the dura mater called

_____ .

12. Identify the labeled parts on this axial section through the region of the midventricular level (Figs. 22-5 and 22-6)

A. _____

B. _____

C. _____

D. _____

E. _____

F. _____

G. _____

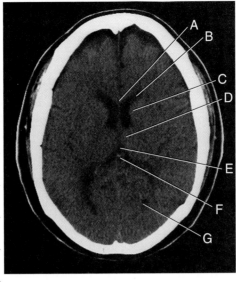

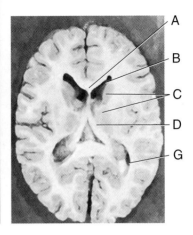

Fig. 22-5. Structure identification on an axial CT scan at midventricular level.

Fig. 22-6. Brain tissue specimen, midventricular level.

13. Identify the labeled parts on this axial section through the level of the middle third ventricle (Figs. 22-7 and 22-8):

A. _____

B. _____

C. _____

D. _____

E. _____

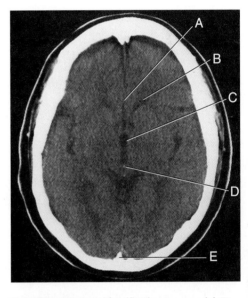

Fig. 22-7. Structure identification on an axial CT scan at mid-third ventricle level.

22

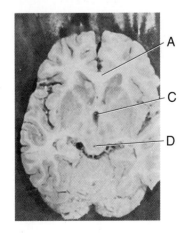

Fig. 22-8. Brain tissue specimen, mid-third ventricle level.

REVIEW EXERCISE D: Thoracic CT and Sectional Anatomy of the Chest (see textbook pp. 743-746)

Positioning and Procedures for Thoracic CT

1. How are the arms positioned for a CT scan of the chest?

    _____

2. Is the patient in a prone or supine position for a routine CT examination of the thorax?

    _____

3. What is the most common slice thickness range for a routine CT study of the chest?

    _____

4. If a small pulmonary lesion is suspected, slice thickness will often be reduced to

    _____ .

5. During volume scanning of the chest, the patient is required to hold his or her breath for a minimum of

    _____ .

6. Which of the following is *not* a pathologic indicator for thoracic CT?

    A. Hilar lesion   E. Pericardial disease

    B. Aneurysm   F. Evaluation of pulmonary nodules

    C. Abscess of thorax   G. All of the above are common indicators

    D. Cardiac disease

7. **Situation:** A mass seen on a thoracic CT study reveals a mass in the lungs. The attenuation of this mass is slightly above water (O). Which one of the following pathologic indicators would be most likely?

    A. Solid pulmonary nodule   C. Bronchogenic cyst

    B. Lung carcinoma   D. Pulmonary calcification

8. **Situation:** A patient with a clinical history of carcinoma of the lung comes to the radiology department for a CT of the thorax. Which one of the following scan ranges would be performed for this patient?

    A. From apex of lung to diaphragm   C. From apex of lung to left colic flexure

    B. From apex of lung to liver   D. From apex of lung to adrenal glands

9. Helical CT scanning uses a _____ breathing technique during CT of the thorax.

10. What is the name of the region located between the ascending aorta and the pulmonary artery?

    _____

Sectional Anatomy of the Thorax: Identify the anatomy on these axial sections of the thorax at 10 mm-slice thickness obtained after bolus injections of iodinated contrast media. The patient's right is to your left as with conventional radiography.

11. Axial section through upper thorax at level of approximately T3 (sternal notch; Fig. 22-9). Parts *A, B, D,* and *E* represent veins and arteries of the lower neck and upper thorax just superior to the arch of the aorta. Parts *F* and *G* are well-known portions of the upper digestive tract and respiratory system that you should be able to identify by their relative locations.

A. _____ vein

B. _____ artery

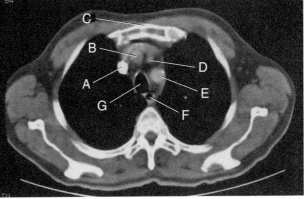

C. _____

D. _____ artery

E. _____ artery

F. _____

G. _____

Fig. 22-9. Axial section through upper thorax at level of about T3.

12. Which one of the following structures is considered to be most posterior (as seen in Fig. 22-9)?

A. Esophagus   C. Left brachiocephalic vein

B. Trachea   D. Left common carotid artery

13. Axial section through approximate level of the carina (Fig. 22-10). Identify labeled structures *A* through *H*, which represent major vessels and bony structures of the chest:

A. _____

B. _____

C. _____

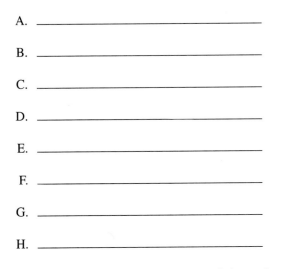

D. _____

E. _____

F. _____

G. _____

H. _____

14. Which one of the following structures is located most anterior (as seen in Fig. 22-10)?

Fig. 22-10. Axial section through level of carina.

A. Superior vena cava   C. Descending aorta

B. Carina   D. Ascending aorta

15. Axial section through the base of the heart (Fig. 22-11). Identify labeled structures *A* through *H*, which represent the four chambers of the heart and other thoracic vessels and structures seen at this level:

A. _____

B. _____

C. _____

D. _____

E. _____

F. _____

G. _____

H. _____

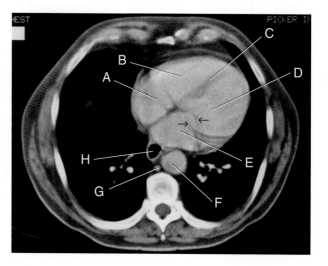

Fig. 22-11. Axial section through four chambers of the heart.

16. How can you determine whether structure *H* is the esophagus or the trachea?

_____

17. The valve between heart chambers D and E is the _____ valve (see arrows).

18. Which chamber of the heart is located closest to the spine? _____

REVIEW EXERCISE E: Abdominal and Pelvic CT and Sectional Anatomy (see textbook pp. 747-752)

1. True/False: The number of ERCP and IVU procedures performed has been greatly reduced because of the superior contrast enhancement of CT examinations of the abdomen.

2. True/False: Pregnancy is not a contraindication for CT of the abdomen.

3. For most routine CT studies of the abdomen or pelvis, a slice thickness of _____ mm is often employed.

    A. 10 to 15   C. 7 to 10

    B. 20   D. 25 to 30

4. True/False: Oral or rectal contrast media are generally required for most abdomen and pelvis CT procedures.

5. Prior to a CT procedure of the abdomen and pelvis, oral contrast media must be ingested:

    A. The night before the exam   C. Immediately before the exam

    B. 1 hour prior to the exam   D. All of the above

6. What concentration of barium sulfate must be used for a CT procedure?

    A. 1% to 3%   C. 10% to 20%

    B. 5% to 8%   D. 30% to 40%

7. What type of artifact may be produced if there is a delay in imaging following the ingestion of barium sulfate?

    A. Ring artifact   C. Signal loss artifact

    B. Streak artifact   D. Ghosting artifact

8. Which of the abdominal CT procedures requires the use of intravenous contrast media?

A. Liver   C. Spleen

B. Pancreas   D. All of the above

9. If the abdomen only is the area of interest, scanning generally begins at the level of the

(A) _____ and continues inferiorly to the level of the (B) _____ .

10. If the pelvis is the area of interest, scanning begins at the level of the (A) _____ and

continues to the (B) _____ .

11. What is the purpose of the insertion of a tampon for CT scans of the female pelvis and lower abdomen?

_____

12. What are breathing requirements for volume (spiral) type scanning of the abdomen?

_____

13. **Situation:** During a helical CT of the abdomen, a 15-mm couch movement per second with a slice collimation of 10 mm is used. Calculate the pitch ratio for this study.

_____

14. **Situation:** A patient with a clinical history of pancreatic cancer comes to CT for a study of the abdomen. What slice thickness should be used for this study at the level of the pancreas?

A. 5 to 8 mm   C. 10 mm

B. 2 to 3 mm   D. 1 to 1.5 mm

Sectional Anatomy of the Abdomen and Pelvis: The following CT images are 10-mm slice thickness. An intravenous contrast medium was given to enhance vascular structures, as well as oral contrast for the GI tract. The pelvis CT images may also include the use of rectal contrast media.

15. Axial section through the level of the pancreatic tail (Fig. 22-12). Identify labeled structures *A* through *K*, which represent major vessels and soft-tissue structures of the abdomen:

A. _____

B. _____

C. _____

D. _____

E. _____

F. _____

G. _____

H. _____

I. _____

J. _____

K. _____

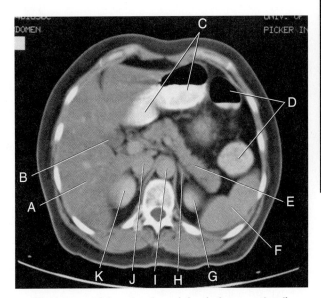

Fig. 22-12. Axial section through level of pancreatic tail.

Questions 16 and 17 relate to structures seen in Fig. 22-12

16. Which two parts of the stomach are indicated by the two lead lines for label C? (Select two of the four choices.)

    A. Pylorus   C. Fundus

    B. Body   D. Cardiac antrum

17. The adrenal glands often appear as an inverted _____ shape seen in sectional images of the abdomen.

18. Axial section through level of the second portion of duodenum (Fig. 22-13). Identify labeled structures *A* through *J*, which represent major vessels and soft-tissue structures of the abdomen:

    A. _____

    B. _____

    C. _____

    D. _____

    E. _____

    F. _____

    G. _____

    H. _____

    I. _____

    J. _____

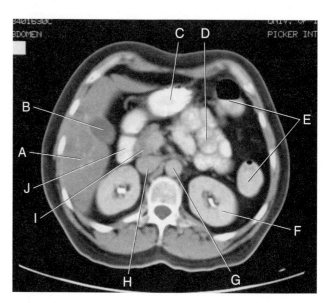

Fig. 22-13. Axial section through level of second portion of duodenum.

19. How can the second portion of the duodenum be distinguished from a tumor in the head of the pancreas as shown in Fig. 22-13?

    _____

20. Axial section through the level 2 cm caudad to the renal pelvis (Fig. 22-14). Identify labeled structures *A* through *I*, which represent major vessels and segments of both the large and small bowel, kidneys, and ureters.

    A. _____

    B. _____

    C. _____

    D. _____

    E. _____

    F. _____

    G. _____

    H. _____

    I. _____

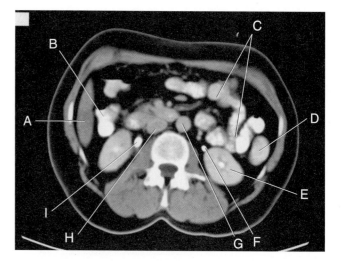

Fig. 22-14. Axial section through the level 2 cm caudad to renal pelvis.

22

21. How can it be determined that the section in Fig. 22-14 is at a level just caudad to the renal pelvis? (HINT: Look at the relationship of the kidneys and ureters.)

_____

22. How can it be determined which is the ascending colon and which is the descending colon on this section (Fig. 22-14)?

_____

23. Axial section through level of the ilium and the rectum (2 cm caudal to iliac crest; Fig. 22-15). Identify labeled structures *A* through *G,* which represent major vessels, soft tissues, and bony structures of the pelvis:

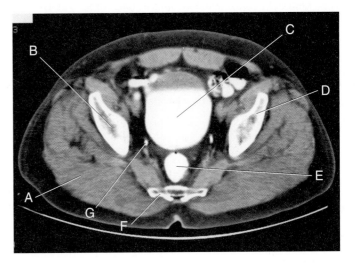

Fig. 22-15. Axial section through level of ilium and rectum.

A. _____

B. _____

C. _____

D. _____

E. _____

F. _____

G. _____

24. Bonus question: What is the name of the double-band muscle located anterior to the bladder?

_____

REVIEW EXERCISE F: Additional and Specialized CT Procedures and CT Terminology (see textbook pp. 753-755)

1. CT scan of the neck for a possible tumor of the nasopharynx will require slice thicknesses of no greater than:

   A. 5 mm   C. 10 mm

   B. 7 mm   D. 1 cm

2. True/False: Air may be injected into the joint for a CT scan of the knee.

3. Common pathologic indications for a CT study of the spine include the following *except:*

   A. Infection   C. Spinal cord deformity

   B. Spinal stenosis   D. Fracture of the vertebrae

4. True/False: Different CT scans can be combined and reformatted to create a three-dimensional image.

5. True/False: Three-dimensional imaging requires a data set created during a volume acquisition.

6. What is the contrast medium of choice for most CT virtual endoscopic procedures? _____

7. What two positions must the patient assume during a virtual colonoscopy? _____

22

8. True/False: Virtual colonoscopy is a more comfortable procedure for the patient as compared with conventional colonoscopy.

9. True/False: The patient/table is stationary during CT fluoroscopy.

10. During CT fluoroscopy, partially reconstructed images are obtained and displayed at a rate of:

    A. 1 to 3 images per second   C. 10 to 12 images per second

    B. 6 to 8 images per second   D. 20 to 25 images per second

11. One of the most common applications for CT fluoroscopy is:

    A. CT myelography   C. Virtual colonoscopy

    B. GI motility studies   D. Biopsies

12. True/False: CT percutaneous biopsies have a higher accuracy rate as compared with surgical biopsies.

13. The success rate for CT percutaneous abscess drainage is approximately:

    A. 10% to 15%   C. 50% to 60%

    B. 20% to 25%   D. 85%

14. Identify the name of the device that houses the CT x-ray tube, detectors, and collimators: _____

15. What is the term for a series of rows and columns of pixels that give form to the digital image? _____

16. What are the terms (more than one answer) for a preliminary image taken prior to CT procedure?

    _____

17. A device that transmits electrical energy and allows continuous rotation of the CT x-ray tube for volumetric

    acquisition is called _____.

18. List the other two terms for "volume scanning":

    A. _____   B. _____

19. _____ controls the **brightness** of a CT reconstructed image within a certain range.

20. _____ controls the gray level or **contrast** of a CT image.

Laboratory Exercises (see textbook pp. 740-753)

Part A of this learning activity needs to be carried out in a special procedures room equipped for whole-body CT. A supervising technologist or instructor should be present for this activity. Part B can be carried out in a classroom or any room in which illuminators and other CT viewing facilities are available.

LABORATORY EXERCISE A: Positioning

Complete the following steps and place a check mark by each when completed.

_____   1.   Review the equipment in the room, noting the location of patient support equipment such as oxygen, suction, the IV pole, and the emergency cart.

_____   2.   Role play using another student as the patient. Prepare the "patient" by explaining the procedure, the breathing instructions they will be given, the sounds they will experience, and what they will see and experience as they are placed into the gantry aperture for the examination.

_____   3.   Place your patient on the table (couch) in a supine position with the arms above the head. Raise the patient and table to the correct height and slowly move into the gantry aperture until the x-ray beam trajectory coincides with the starting scan position for the part being examined. Using the intercom device, talk to the patient from the control console. Finally, remove your patient when the procedure is completed.

_____   4.   Review the controls and monitors at the operator console. Have someone demonstrate the image parameters and the other variables controlled by the technologist and explain how whole body scanning is different from cranial CT scanning.

LABORATORY EXERCISE B: Anatomy Review Using CT Scans

Use CT scans of the thorax (chest), abdomen, and pelvis as provided by your instructor. These may be "hard-copies" recorded on film, or they may be from a PACS and displayed on a monitor. Scans should include normal and abnormal sections displaying obvious pathology.

Locate and identify each of the organs and structures as labeled and identified on similar scans in the workbook and the textbook. (Pay particular attention to those parts you identified on similar scans in your workbook in the preceding Review Exercises D and E.)

_____   1.   Axial sections of the chest

_____   2.   Axial sections of the abdomen

_____   3.   Axial sections of the pelvis

22

Answers to Review Exercises

Review Exercise A: Anatomy of the Central Nervous System

1. A. Brain (encephalon)
   B. Spinal cord (medulla spinalis)
2. A. L1
   B. Conus medullaris
3. A. Neurons
   B. Dendrites
4. A. Dura mater
   B. Arachnoid
   C. Pia mater
   D. Epidural space
   E. Subdural space
   F. Subarachnoid space
5. Venous sinuses
6. A. Frontal lobe
   B. Parietal lobe
   C. Occipital lobe
   D. Temporal lobe
   E. Insula or central lobe
7. A. Cerebrum
   B. Thalamus
   C. Hypothalamus
   D. Cerebellum
   E. Pons
   F. Medulla (medulla oblongata)
8. A. Occipital lobe
   B. Parietal lobe
   C. Frontal lobe
   D. Longitudinal fissure
9. E. Anterior (precentral) central gyrus
   F. Central sulcus
   G. Posterior (post central) central gyrus
10. D. Corpus callosum
11. B. Longitudinal fissure
12. A. Cerebrospinal fluid
    B. CSF
    C. Subarachnoid
    D. Hydrocephalus
13. A. Cisterns
    B. Cistern cerebellomedullaris (Cisterna magna)
14. Brain stem
15. A. Hypothalamus
    B. Pituitary (hypophysis) gland
16. A. Pineal gland
    B. Cerebellum
17. A. Tracts of myelinated axons of nerve cells
    B. Primarily dendrites and cell bodies
18. A. Gray
    B. White
19. A. Infundibulum
    B. Posterior pituitary gland
    C. Optic chiasma
20. A. Midbrain
    B. Pons
    C. Medulla
21. C. Thalamus
22. B. Cerebellum
23. D. Hypothalamus
24. B. Pituitary gland
25. A. Caudate nucleus
    B. Lentiform nucleus
    C. Claustrum
    D. Amygdaloid nucleus
26. A. Lateral
    B. Third
    C. Fourth
    1. Posterior horn
    2. Body
    3. Anterior horn
    4. Interventricular foramen
    5. Cerebral aqueduct
    6. Inferior horn
    7. Lateral recess
    8. Pineal gland
27. A. Olfactory
    B. Optic
    C. Oculomotor
    D. Trochlear
    E. Trigeminal
    F. Abducens
    G. Facial
    H. Acoustic
    I. Glossopharyngeal
    J. Vagus
    K. Spinal accessory
    L. Hypoglossal

Review Exercise B: Basic Principles of Computed Tomography (CT)

1. A. Visualization of anatomic structures with no superimposition
   B. Better contrast resolution between various types of soft tissue
   C. MPR (multiplanar reconstruction)
   D. Manipulation of attenuation data
2. 1. B
   2. A
   3. E
   4. C
   5. C and D
   6. D and E
   7. C
   8. A
   9. D
   10. C and D
   11. D
   12. E
   13. C
3. False (number and arrangement of the detectors)
4. True
5. False (multiple rotations possible)
6. True
7. C. Slip rings
8. D. Low-cost system to operate
9. B. 0.5 mm or higher
10. A. Gantry
    B. Operator control console
    C. Computer
11. Gantry
12. Aperture
13. Cadmium tungstate or rare earth oxide ceramic crystals
14. D. Postpatient collimator
15. D. 262,144
16. A. PACS
17. Attenuation of radiation by a given tissue
18. Volume element
19. Three, two
20. A. Slice thickness
21. B. Isotropic
22. C. Attenuation
23. Lower
24. Attenuation
25. A. Cortical bone: +1000 to +3000
    B. White brain matter: +45
    C. Blood: +20
    D. Fat: −100
    E. Lung tissue: −200
    F. Air: −1000
    G. Water: 0
26. Water
27. A. 1
    B. 2
    C. 3
    D. 1
28. B. Displayed image contrast
29. A. Image brightness
30. Amount of anatomy covered during a particular scan
31. Table speed; slice thickness
32. 2:1 pitch
33. A. Undersampling
34. C. 10-mm couch movement and 20-mm slice thickness

Review Exercise C: Clinical Applications of Head CT and Sectional Anatomy of the Brain

1. B. Scout view
2. 50% to 90%
3. False (4 minutes)
4. False (not able to pass through)
5. True
6. A. Proteins
7. True
8. True
9. A. Brain windows
   B. Bone windows
10. Rotation; tilt
11. Subdural hematoma

22

12. A. Anterior corpus callosum-genu
    B. Anterior horn of left lateral ventricle
    C. Region of caudate nuclei
    D. Region of thalamus
    E. Third ventricle
    F. Pineal gland or body
    G. Posterior horn of left lateral ventricle
13. A. Anterior corpus callosum-genu
    B. Anterior horn of left lateral ventricle (CT only)
    C. Third ventricle
    D. Region of pineal gland
    E. Internal occipital protuberance (CT only)

Review Exercise D: Thoracic CT and Sectional Anatomy of the Chest

Positioning and Procedures for Thoracic CT

1. Elevated above the head
2. Supine position
3. 7 to 10 mm
4. 2 to 3 mm
5. 20 to 30 seconds
6. G. All are common indications
7. C. Bronchogenic cyst
8. D. From apex of lung to adrenal glands
9. Breath hold or single-breath
10. Aortopulmonary window

Sectional Anatomy of the Thorax

11. A. Right brachiocephalic vein
    B. Brachiocephalic artery
    C. Sternum (manubrium)
    D. Left common carotid artery
    E. Left subclavian artery
    F. Esophagus
    G. Trachea
12. A. Esophagus
13. A. Left mainstem bronchus
    B. Descending aorta
    C. T5 vertebra
    D. Esophagus
    E. Carina
    F. Right mainstem bronchus
    G. Superior vena cava
    H. Ascending aorta
14. D. Ascending aorta
15. A. Right atrium
    B. Right ventricle
    C. Interventricular septum
    D. Left ventricle
    E. Left atrium
    F. Descending aorta
    G. Azygos vein
    H. Esophagus

16. This level (through the base of the heart) is below (or inferior to) the carina, so H couldn't be the trachea.
17. Mitral
18. Left atrium

Review Exercise E: Abdominal and Pelvic CT and Sectional Anatomy of Abdomen and Pelvis

1. True
2. False (is a contraindication). Although the radiologist may still order CT if no other imaging modality will produce the needed diagnosis.
3. C. 7 to 10
4. True
5. D. All of the above
6. A. 1 to 3%
7. B. Streak artifact
8. D. All of the above
9. A. Diaphragm
   B. Iliac crest
10. A. Iliac crest
    B. Symphysis pubis
11. Added contrast and localization of the vaginal region
12. With volume acquisition, a single breath hold of 20 to 30 seconds is required.
13. 1.5:1.0
14. A. 5 to 8 mm

Sectional Anatomy of the Abdomen and Pelvis

15. A. Right lobe of the liver (posterior segment)
    B. Gallbladder
    C. Stomach
    D. Colon (descending)
    E. Tail of pancreas
    F. Spleen
    G. Upper lobe of left kidney
    H. Left adrenal gland
    I. Aorta
    J. Inferior vena cava
    K. Upper lobe of right kidney
16. A and B (pylorus and body)
17. "V"
18. A. Right lobe of liver
    B. Gallbladder
    C. Stomach
    D. Jejunum
    E. Colon (descending)
    F. Left kidney
    G. Abdominal aorta
    H. Inferior vena cava

    I. Head of pancreas
    J. Second portion of duodenum
19. Give the patient oral contrast media to increase attenuation of the duodenum
20. A. Lower portion of right lobe of liver
    B. Ascending colon
    C. Jejunum
    D. Descending colon
    E. Left kidney
    F. Left ureter
    G. Abdominal aorta
    H. Inferior vena cava
    I. Right ureter
21. The ureters are seen in cross-section totally separate from the kidneys. (Above the renal pelvis ureters would not be visible, and at level of the renal pelvis ureters and kidneys would appear connected.)
22. Ascending would be on patient's right (side of liver) and descending would be on left.
23. A. Gluteus maximus muscle
    B. Right ilium
    C. Urinary bladder (with contrast media)
    D. Left ilium
    E. Rectum (with barium)
    F. Sacrum
    G. Right ureter
24. Rectus abdominis muscle

Review Exercise F: Additional and Specialized CT Procedures and CT Terminology

1. A. 5 mm
2. True
3. C. Spinal cord deformity
4. False
5. True
6. Air
7. Prone and supine
8. True
9. True
10. B. 6 to 8 images per second
11. D. Biopsies
12. True
13. D. 85%
14. Gantry
15. Matrix
16. Scanogram, topogram, or scout
17. Slip rings
18. A. Helical scanning
    B. Spiral scanning
19. Window level (WL)
20. Window width (WW)

22

SELF-TEST

This self-test should be taken only after completing all of the readings, review exercises, and laboratory activities for a particular section. The purpose of this test is not only to provide a good learning exercise but also to serve as a good indicator of what your final evaluation exam will be. It is strongly suggested that if you do not get at least a 90% to 95% grade on this self-test, you review those areas in which you missed questions before going to your instructor for the final evaluation exam for this chapter. (There are 100 questions or blanks—each is worth 1 point.)

1. Which generation of CT scanner uses a pencil-thin x-ray beam and a single detector?

    A. First-generation   C. Third-generation

    B. Second-generation   D. Fourth-generation

2. Which generation of CT scanner allows continuous volume-type scanning? (There may be more than one correct answer.)

    A. First-generation   C. Third-generation

    B. Second-generation   D. Fourth-generation

3. Which devices in the volume CT scanners allow continual tube rotation in the same direction? _____

4. CT can detect tissue density differences as low as:

    A. 1%   C. 10%

    B. 5%   D. 20%

5. Which device controls slice thickness in a CT image? _____

6. What must be done to the numeric data (CT numbers) to create the displayed CT image?

    _____

7. The three major components of the scan unit are:

    A. _____   B. _____   C. _____

8. Each tiny picture element in the display matrix is called a(n) _____ .

9. Which of the following parameters *cannot* be varied by appropriate manipulation at the operator console?

    A. kV   D. Vertical adjustment of table height

    B. Scan time   E. Thickness of slice

    C. Pitch selections

10. What is the name of the three-dimensional element that provides height, width, and depth to the display matrix of the digital image?

    A. Pixel   C. Image volume

    B. Voxel   D. Isotrophic data set

11. True/False: Artifacts due to patient motion are reduced with volume CT scanners as compared with earlier scanners.

12. Current multislice CT scanners are capable of producing up to _____ slices per x-ray tube rotation.

    A. 10   C. 35

    B. 16   D. 40

13. What does the detector actually measure in a CT system? _____

14. What substance serves as the baseline for CT numbers? _____

15. What is the CT number for the substance described in question 14? _____

16. What is the CT number for fat?

    A. − 100   C. + 100

    B. − 200   D. + 250

17. Pitch is defined as a ratio between table speed and:

    A. Number of tube rotations   C. Slice thickness

    B. Size of total tissue acquisition   D. Tissue attenuation

18. Which one of the following pitch ratios represents "undersampling"?

    A. 1:1   C. 0.5:1

    B. 2:1   D. 0.7:1

19. True/False: CT exceeds the contrast resolution seen on a conventional radiograph.

20. Contrast media will not ordinarily cross the _____ barrier.

21. Which one of the following pathologic indications does *not* apply to head CT?

    A. Brain neoplasm   D. Trauma

    B. Brain atrophy   E. All of the above apply

    C. Multiple sclerosis

22. Considering the blood-brain barrier phenomenon, which of the following pathologic indicators would require the use of contrast media during a CT scan? (There may be more than one correct answer.)

    A. Hydrocephalus   D. Epidural hematoma

    B. Possible neoplasia   E. Brain tumor

    C. Subdural hematoma

23. A. The parts of the neuron that conduct impulses toward the cell body are called _____ .

    B. The part that conducts impulses away from the cell body is the _____ .

24. Three protective membranes that cover or enclose the entire central nervous system are collectively called:

    _____

25. The three specific membranes from question 24 are called (starting externally):

    A. _____   B. _____   C. _____

26. The various layers of the membranes just discussed have specific spaces of various sizes between these layers. Each has a specific name. Identify these various membrane layers and their associated spaces on Fig. 22-16:

A. _____

B. _____

C. _____

D. _____

E. _____

F. _____

G. _____

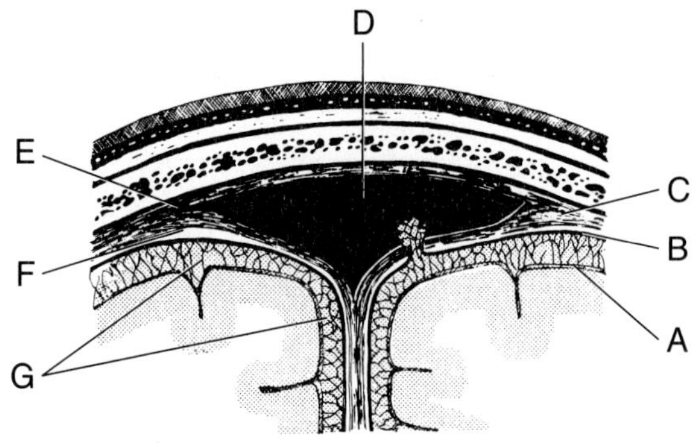

Fig. 22-16. Meninges and meningeal spaces.

27. Which of the spaces in question 26 is normally filled with cerebrospinal fluid? _____

28. Match the following structures to the correct division of the brain.

_____ A. Pons   1. Forebrain

_____ B. Cerebellum   2. Midbrain

_____ C. Cerebrum   3. Hindbrain

_____ D. Thalamus

_____ E. Medulla

29. The largest division of the brain is the _____ .

30. The right and left cerebral hemispheres are separated by a deep fissure called the _____ .

31. The fibrous band of white tissue deep within this fissure connecting the right and left cerebral hemispheres is

called the _____ .

32. What is the name of the tissue found within the fissure mentioned in question 30? _____

33. Which of the following ventricles are located in the upper aspect of the cerebral hemispheres?

A. Lateral ventricles   C. Third ventricle

B. Fourth ventricle   D. Cisterna magna

34. The diamond-shaped fourth ventricle connects inferiorly with a wide portion of subarachnoid space called the:

A. Interventricular foramen   C. Cisterna cerebellomedullaris

B. Lateral recesses   D. Cisterna pontis

22

35. Identify the ventricles, their parts, and their associated structures as labeled on both the lateral and top-view drawings (Figs. 22-17 and 22-18):

Ventricles

A. _____

B. _____

C. _____

Connecting ducts

a. _____

b. _____

c. _____

Parts of lateral ventricles

1. _____

2. _____

3. _____

4. _____

Associated structure (only in Fig. 22-17)

5. _____

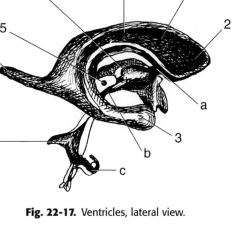

Fig. 22-17. Ventricles, lateral view.

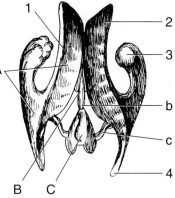

Fig. 22-18. Ventricles, superior view.

36. The condition known as _____ results from abnormal accumulation of cerebrospinal fluid

within the _____ .

37. Enlarged regions of the subarachnoid space are called _____ .

38. Identify the four lobes of the cerebrum as labeled on Fig. 22-19:

A. _____

B. _____

C. _____

D. _____

E. The fifth lobe, which is more centrally located and not shown on this drawing, is called the

_____ .

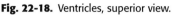

Fig. 22-19. Four lobes of the cerebrum.

39. Identify each of the following terms as either gray matter or white matter brain structures:

     _____ A. Cerebral cortex   1. Gray matter

     _____ B. Axons (fibrous parts of neuron)   2. White matter

     _____ C. Corpus callosum

     _____ D. Thalamus

     _____ E. Centrum semiovale

     _____ F. Cerebral nuclei

Questions 40 through 43 refer to anatomy as seen on axial thoracic CT sections (*see textbook pp. 744-755*)

40. The brachiocephalic artery would be best demonstrated on an axial section at the level of the:
    A. Sternal notch   C. Body portion of manubrium
    B. Inferior portion of manubrium   D. Carina

41. The right internal jugular vein would only be clearly seen on axial sections at the level of the:
    A. Sternal notch   C. Carina
    B. Inferior portion of manubrium   D. Base of the heart

42. The ascending aorta would be clearly seen on axial sections at the level of the:
    A. Superior portion of manubrium   D. Carina
    B. Sternal notch   E. All of the above
    C. Aortopulmonary window

43. The right hemidiaphragm only would generally be seen on axial sections at the level of the:
    A. Base of the heart   D. Aortopulmonary window
    B. 2 cm below the base of the heart   E. None of the above
    C. Carina

44. The space between the ascending and descending aorta is called _____ .

45. Which one of the following structures is considered to be most anterior at the level of the carina?
    A. Ascending aorta   D. Left mainstem bronchus
    B. Descending aorta   E. Azygos vein
    C. Carina

46. Which chamber of the heart is considered to be most posterior at the level of the base of the heart?
    A. Right atrium   C. Left atrium
    B. Right ventricle   D. Left ventricle

47. Which of the following is *not* a pathologic indication for CT of the thorax?
    A. Evaluation of pulmonary nodules   C. Hilar lesions
    B. Aneurysms   D. Mitral valve prolapse

22

48.   A slice thickness is commonly used for a routine CT scan of the thorax.

    A. 10 mm   B. 5 mm   C. 2 mm   D. 10 cm

Questions 49 through 53 refer to anatomy as seen on the axial abdomen and pelvic CT sections (*see textbook pp. 747-752*)

49.   The uncinate process refers to:

    A. A section of the liver located posteriorly and inferiorly

    B. A hooklike process of the spleen as seen lying next to the duodenum

    C. A process of the gallbladder seen only in the appropriate axial section

    D. The hooklike extension of the head of the pancreas

50.   The right lobe of the liver is demonstrated on axial sections at the same level(s) of the:

    A. Pancreatic tail   C. Uncinate process of pancreas

    B. Midportion of the kidneys   D. All of the above

51.   The gallbladder is visualized on the same axial level as the:

    A. Renal pelves of kidneys   C. Right lobe of the liver

    B. Uncinate process of the pancreas   D. All of the above

52.   The prostate gland is best visualized at the same axial section level as the:

    A. Ischial rami   C. Urinary bladder

    B. Acetabular roof   D. Symphysis pubis

53.   Which one of the following structures is considered to be most anterior (at the level of the femoral heads)?

    A. Rectum   C. Urinary bladder

    B. Seminal vesicles   D. Coccyx

54.   A common slice thickness for abdominal scanning is:

    A. 10 cm   B. 10 mm   C. 1 cm   D. 5 mm

55.   Streak artifacts for CT of the abdomen are most likely to occur when:

    A. Patient has metallic parts such as a hip prosthesis

    B. High concentration of a large bolus of barium is present with a low concentration of water

    C. Low concentration of barium (too diluted with water) is present

    D. Answers A and B

56.   The first slice for an abdomen-only CT scan is commonly taken at the level of:

    A. First lumbar vertebra   C. Xiphoid process

    B. Inferior rib margin   D. Iliac crest

57.   True/False: The use of CT has greatly reduced use of the ERCP as a common standard diagnostic procedure for evaluating the biliary ducts.

58.   True/False: The use of water-soluble contrast agents rather than barium sulfate suspensions for GI tract radiography is desirable because they tend to slow peristaltic action.

59.   True/False: Because of the relatively short exposure times, patients are not required to hold their breath during CT exposures of the abdomen.

60. True/False: The use of both oral and/or rectal contrast media is essential for most CT abdominal and pelvic exams.

61. True/False: Contrast media are injected intravenously in a similar manner (but with greater speed) to excretory urography to visualize structures within the mediastinum for thoracic CT.

62. For a volume CT scan of the thorax, the patient must be able to hold his or her breath at least:

    A. 5 seconds   C. 20 seconds

    B. 10 seconds   D. 2 minutes

63. Typical slice thickness for a spine CT ranges between:

    A. 3 to 5 mm   C. 10 to 15 mm

    B. 7 to 10 mm   D. 15 to 20 mm

64. A virtual CT colonoscopy requires the use of _____ as a contrast medium.

    A. Barium sulfate   C. Air

    B. Iodinated rectal contrast   D. All of the above

65. True/False: Special filters can be used during CT fluoroscopy to reduce patient skin dose.

66. _____ is a method by which images acquired in the axial plane may be reconstructed in the coronal or sagittal plane.

67. _____ controls the gray level of an image (the contrast).

22

CHAPTER 23

Additional Diagnostic Procedures

This chapter discusses those additional diagnostic imaging procedures that are less common in most radiology departments. Arthrograms, sialograms, myelograms, and conventional tomograms are largely being replaced with other imaging modalities such as computed tomography (CT) or magnetic resonance imaging (MRI). However, in some departments, these procedures are still being performed in sufficient numbers that technologists need to be familiar with them so that they can perform them when requested.

The anatomy for these procedures has been studied in previous chapters; this chapter therefore covers only the procedures themselves and the related positioning. The exception to this is the anatomy of the female reproductive organs as described in the section on hysterosalpingography.

CHAPTER OBJECTIVES

After you have successfully completed the activities of this chapter, you will be able to:

Arthrography

_____ 1. Identify the purpose, indications, patient preparation, equipment, general procedure, and the positioning routines related to knee arthrography.

_____ 2. Identify the purpose, indications, patient preparation, equipment, general procedure, and the positioning and filming sequence related to shoulder arthrography.

Hysterosalpingography

_____ 1. Identify specific aspects of the female reproductive system.

_____ 2. Identify the purpose, indications, patient preparation, equipment, general procedure, and the positioning routines related to hysterosalpingography.

Orthoroentgenography

_____ 1. Define _orthoroentgenography_ and the purpose of this procedure.

_____ 2. Identify the specific positioning and procedure for lower and upper limb orthoroentgenography.

Myelography

_____ 1. Identify the purpose, indications, contraindications, equipment, and general procedure related to myelography.

_____ 2. Identify positioning routines performed for lumbar, thoracic, and cervical myelography.

Sialography

_____ 1. Identify major aspects of the salivary glands.

_____ 2. Identify the purpose, indications, patient preparation, equipment, general procedure, and the positioning routines related to sialography.

Conventional Tomography

_____ 1. Define the specific terms associated with conventional tomography.

_____ 2. Identify the controls and variables that are common features on conventional tomographic units.

_____ 3. Identify the three influencing and controlling factors related to tomographic blur.

_____ 4. Describe briefly the two variations of conventional tomography, including autotomography (breathing technique) and pantomography (Panorex).

_____ 5. Demonstrate the principles and controlling factors of conventional tomography in laboratory exercises.

Bone Densitometry

_____ 1. List the major components of bone and their function.

_____ 2. List common clinical and pathologic indicators for osteoporosis.

_____ 3. Define and list the risk factors for fracture risk and osteoporosis.

_____ 4. List the World Health Organization (WHO) criteria for the diagnosis of osteoporosis.

_____ 5. List and describe the two general types of agents approved by the FDA for the treatment and prevention of osteoporosis and the specific drugs approved under each type.

_____ 6. Identify the three most common types of equipment, methods, and techniques for determining bone mineral density.

_____ 7. Define and describe the meaning of the two terms *DXA precision* and *DXA accuracy* as used in the performance of bone densitometry procedures.

Learning Exercises

The following review exercises should be completed only after careful study of the associated pages in the textbook as indicated by each exercise. Answers to each review exercise are given at the end of the review exercises.

REVIEW EXERCISE A: Arthrography (see textbook pp. 758-762)

1. What classifications of joints are studied with arthrography? _____

2. Other than conventional radiography of synovial joints (e.g., arthrography), what imaging procedure is preferred by physicians for studying synovial joints? _____

3. List the three common forms of knee injury that require arthrography:

    A. _____

    B. _____

    C. _____

4. Give an example of nontraumatic pathology of the knee joint indicating arthrography. _____

5. What are the two primary contraindications for arthrography of any joint?

    _____

6. True/False: An arthrogram must be approached as a sterile procedure; proper skin prep and sterility must be maintained.

7. True/False: Once the contrast medium is introduced into the knee joint, the knee must *not* be flexed or exercised.

8.   A.   For a knee arthrogram, a _____ -ml syringe is used with a _____ -gauge needle to draw up _____ ml of positive contrast medium for injection.

     B.   If dual-contrast media are used, a _____ -ml syringe is used to introduce the negative contrast media into the joint.

9.   List the two types of contrast media used for a knee arthrogram:

     A.   _____

     B.   _____

10.   List the two projections for conventional "overhead" projections used for knee arthrography:

     A.   _____

     B.   _____

11.   A.   How much is the limb rotated between fluoroscopic spot films of the knee joint? _____

     B.   How many exposures of each meniscus are generally taken with this method? _____

12.   A.   How many exposures are taken of each meniscus during horizontal beam arthrography of the knee?

         _____

     B.   How many degrees of rotation of the leg between exposures? _____

13.   What four aspects of shoulder anatomy are demonstrated with shoulder arthrography?

     A.   _____   C.   _____

     B.   _____   D.   _____

14.   What is the general name for the conjoined tendons of the four major shoulder muscles? _____

15.   What type of needle is commonly used for shoulder arthrograms? _____

16.   A.   For a single-contrast study of the shoulder joint, how much positive contrast medium is commonly used?

         _____

     B.   For a dual contrast study, _____ ml of positive contrast medium and _____ ml of negative medium is used (e.g., room air).

17.   List the six projections frequently taken during a shoulder arthrogram:

     A.   _____   D.   _____

     B.   _____   E.   _____

     C.   _____   F.   _____

18.   Caudad angulations of the CR of _____ ° to _____ ° may be used for the AP projections of the shoulder.

23

REVIEW EXERCISE B: Hysterosalpingography (see textbook pp. 763-765)

1. The hysterosalpingogram is a radiographic study of the _____ and _____ .

2. The uterus is situated between the _____ posteriorly and the _____ anteriorly.

3. List the four divisions of the uterus:

    A. _____

    B. _____

    C. _____

    D. _____

4. The largest division of the uterus is the _____ .

5. The distal aspect of the uterus extending to the vagina is the _____ .

6. List the three layers of tissue that form the uterus (from the innermost to the outermost layer):

    A. _____

    B. _____

    C. _____

7. Which of the following terms is not an aspect of the uterine tube?
    A. Cornu   C. Isthmus
    B. Ampulla   D. Infundibulum

8. True/False: Fertilization of the ovum occurs in the uterine tube.

9. True/False: The distal portion of the uterine tube opens into the peritoneal cavity.

10. Which of the following terms is used to describe the "degree of openness" of the uterine tube?
    A. Stenosis   C. Atresia
    B. Patency   D. Gauge

11. The most common pathologic indication for the hysterosalpingogram (HSG) is:

    _____ .

12. In addition to the answer for question 11, what are two other pathologic indications for HSG?

    A. _____

    B. _____

13. List the three common types of lesions that can be demonstrated during a hysterosalpingogram:

    A. _____

    B. _____

    C. _____

14. The contrast medium preferred by most radiologists for a hysterosalpingogram is:

    A. Water-soluble, iodinated   C. Oxygen

    B. Oil-based, iodinated   D. Nitrogen

15. What device may be needed to aid the insertion and fixation of the cannula or catheter during the

    hysterosalpingogram? _____

16. To help facilitate the flow of contrast media into the uterine cavity, which position is the patient placed into

    following the injection of contrast media? _____

17. In addition to the supine position, what two other positions may be imaged to adequately visualize pertinent
    anatomy for an HSG?

    A. _____

    B. _____

18. Where is the CR centered for overhead projections taken during an HSG using a 24 × 30 cm (10 × 12 inch) image
    receptor?

    A. At level of ASIS   C. Iliac crest

    B. Symphysis pubis   D. 2 inches (5 cm) superior to symphysis pubis

REVIEW EXERCISE C: Myelography (see textbook pp. 766-770)

1. Myelography is a radiographic study of the:

   A. _____

   B. _____

2. List the four common lesions or pathologic indications demonstrated during myelography:

   A. _____   C. _____

   B. _____   D. _____

3. Of the four pathologic indications just mentioned, which is the most common for myelography? _____

4. True/False: Myelography of the cervical and thoracic spinal regions is most common.

5. List the four common contraindications for myelography:

   A. _____   C. _____

   B. _____   D. _____

6. What type of radiographic table must be used for myelography? _____

7. To reduce patient anxiety, a sedative is usually administered _____ hour(s) before the procedure.

8. Into what space is the contrast medium introduced with myelography? _____

9.   List the two common puncture sites for contrast media injection during myelography:

A.   _____

B.   _____

10.   Which one of the puncture sites from question 9 is preferred? _____

11.   What is the patient's general body position for each of the following punctures? (NOTE: There may be more than one acceptable answer for each.)

A.   Lumbar _____

B.   Cervical _____

12.   Why is a large positioning block placed under the abdomen for a lumbar puncture in the prone position?

_____

13.   Which type of contrast medium is most commonly used for myelography? _____

14.   The contrast medium in question 13 will provide good radiopacity up to _____ following injection.

A.   20 minutes   C.   1 hour

B.   30 minutes   D.   8 hours

15.   What dosage range of contrast medium is ideal for myelography?

A.   8 to 10 ml   C.   6 to 17 ml

B.   20 to 30 ml   D.   Approximately 1 ml

16.   Indicate the correct sequence of events for a myelogram by numbering the following steps in order (from 1 through 8):

_____   A.   Introduce needle into subarachnoid space

_____   B.   Collect CSF and send to laboratory

_____   C.   Take overhead radiographic images

_____   D.   Explain the procedure to the patient

_____   E.   Introduce the contrast medium

_____   F.   Have patient sign informed consent form

_____   G.   Take fluoroscopic spot images

_____   H.   Prepare patient's skin for puncture

17.   Which position is performed to demonstrate the region of C7 to T4 during a cervical myelogram?

_____

18.   Why should the patient's head and neck remain hyperextended during cervical myelography?

_____

19. True/False: Generally, AP supine, PA prone, or horizontal beam lateral projections are not taken during thoracic spine myelography.

20. Complete the following for suggested basic routine projections (following fluoroscopy and spot-filming) for the different levels of the spine:

PROJECTION/POSITION   *LEVEL OF CR*

   1. Cervical region   A. _____

                             B. _____

   2. Thoracic region   A. _____

                             B. _____

                             C. _____

   3. Lumbar region   A. _____

21. True/False: Myelography is largely being replaced by MRI and CT.

REVIEW EXERCISE D: Sialography (see textbook pp. 771-773)

1. List the three pairs of salivary glands:

    A. _____

    B. _____

    C. _____

2. Which is the largest of the salivary glands? _____

3. Which is the smallest of the salivary glands? _____

4. List the two terms for the duct that carries saliva from the parotid gland to the oral cavity:

    A. _____

    B. _____

5. Which one of the following is *not* a correct term for the duct leading from the submandibular gland to the oral cavity?

    A. Wharton's duct   C. Submandibular duct

    B. Submaxillary duct   D. Bartholin's duct

6. The 12 small ducts leading from the sublingual glands to the oral cavity are called:

    A. Wharton's ducts   C. Stensen's ducts

    B. Ducts of Rivinus   D. Accessory salivary ducts

7. What is the term for the center, vertical fold membrane located under the tongue? _____

8. Identify the salivary glands and associated ducts labeled on Fig. 23-1:

   A. _____ (a duct)

   B. _____

   C. _____ (a duct)

   D. _____ (a duct)

   E. _____

   F. _____

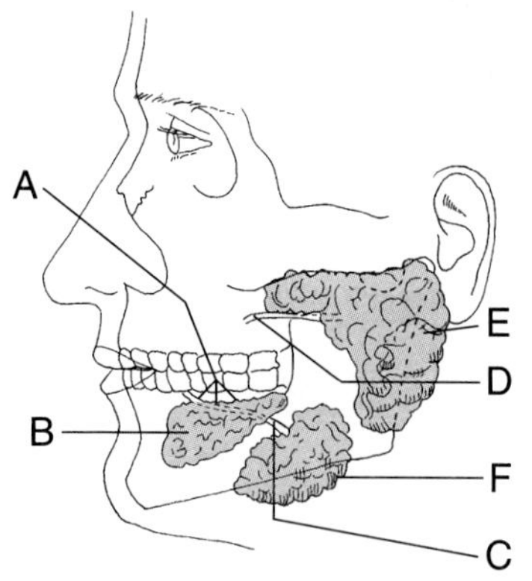

Fig. 23-1. Salivary glands and associated ducts.

9. List the three most common pathologic indications that can lead to an obstruction of the salivary ductal system:

   A. _____

   B. _____

   C. _____

10. Sialectasia is:

    A. Dilation of the salivary duct   C. Inflammation of the salivary gland

    B. Stricture of the salivary duct   D. Inability to produce saliva

11. Why is the patient given a lemon slice to suck at the onset of the sialogram?

    _____

12. What is the name of the special device that helps locate the opening into the salivary duct? _____

13. List the two devices used to cannulate a salivary duct once the duct is located to introduce the contrast media.

    A. _____   B. _____

14. If conventional tomography is used during a sialogram, _____ (**oil-based** or **water-soluble**) contrast medium is recommended.

15. If calculi in one of the salivary ducts are suspected, _____ (**oil-based** or **water-soluble**) contrast media should be used.

16. On the average, how much contrast medium is injected to fill a salivary duct? _____

17. Which one of the following imaging modalities is not used during a sialogram?

    A. Conventional radiography   C. CT

    B. Sonography   D. Digital fluoroscopy

18. Which one of the following imaging positions/projections is not usually performed during a sialogram?

    A. Superoinferior projection   C. AP/PA projection

    B. Lateral position   D. Lateral oblique position

REVIEW EXERCISE E: Orthoroentgenography (see textbook pp. 774-776)

1. Why is orthoroentgenography more commonly used in long bone measurements rather than CT?

    _____

2. What is the literal meaning of the term *orthoroentgenogram?*

    _____

3. Why should separate projections be taken of limb joints rather than including the entire extremity on a single projection?

    _____

4. When performing an orthoroentgenographic procedure, what device needs to be placed on top of the table next to

    the affected limb? _____

5. What is the name of the surgical procedure that shortens a limb by fusing the epiphyses? _____

6. Which three joints are included on one image receptor for a long bone study of the lower limb?

    _____

7. True/False: Both right and left lower limbs can be placed on the same radiograph for a long bone study.

8. True/False: For a bilateral study, all three joints of both lower limbs can be placed on the same 35- × 43-cm (14- × 17-inch) IR.

9. If both lower limbs are radiographed together on one image receptor, why should two rulers be used with one under each limb rather than placing one midway between the two limbs?

    _____

10. True/False: For a long bone study of the upper limb, all three projections must be taken with the IR placed in the Bucky tray.

11. True/False: The wrist is examined in the pronated position (PA) for a long bone study of the upper limb.

12. True/False: The proximal humerus must be rotated internally for the shoulder projection taken during upper limb orthoroentgenography.

REVIEW EXERCISE F: Conventional Tomography (see textbook pp. 777-780)

1. Define each of the following terms in short, concise answers:

    A. Tomograph _____

    B. Fulcrum _____

    C. Fulcrum level _____

    D. Objective (focal) plane _____

    E. Sectional thickness _____

    F. Exposure angle _____

    G. Tube movement (shift) _____

      H.   Amplitude ——————————————————————————————————————

      I.   Blur ——

      J.   Blur margin ———

2.   Which locks on the x-ray tube must be unlocked during linear tomography? ————————————————

3.   True/False: The Bucky tray lock must be securely locked prior to a tomographic exposure.

4.   True/False: Anatomy at the fulcrum level becomes blurred and difficult to see on a radiograph

5.   List four common adjustments or settings found on the tomographic control panel:

      A. —————————————————————————————

      B. —————————————————————————————

      C. —————————————————————————————

      D. —————————————————————————————

6.   True/False: Objects closer to the objective plane will experience maximum blurring.

7.   Briefly describe the tomographic blurring principle. (Why, or how, does blurring of some objects occur while others remain in sharp focus?)

      ——

      ——

8.   List the three factors that determine the amount of blurring:

      A. —————————————————————————————

      B. —————————————————————————————

      C. —————————————————————————————

9.   True/False: As the exposure angle decreases, slice thickness also decreases (becomes thinner).

10.   True/False: As the distance from the image receptor increases, object blurring increases.

11.   To gain maximum blurring of the body of the sternum during tomography, it should be placed

      ————————————————— to tube movement.

      A. Parallel   C. Diagonally

      B. Perpendicular   D. 5° angle

12.   Which of the following exposure angles would produce the least amount of blurring outside of the objective plane?

      A. 10°   C. 5°

      B. 20°   D. 40°

13.   Which of the following exposure angles would produce the greatest amount of blurring outside of the objective plane?

      A. 10°   C. 5°

      B. 8°   D. 20°

14.   True/False: The human eye accepts a certain degree of blurring as normal, making the actual amount of blurring somewhat subjective.

15. A tomographic principle in which the anatomic structure moves but the image receptor/tube remain stationary is

    called _____ . (HINT: It is used in certain lateral spine and sternum projections to blur out overlying structures)

16. What is the most common application for pantotomography? _____

17. What device minimizes penumbra blurring during a pantotomographic procedure? _____

REVIEW EXERCISE G: Bone Densitometry (see textbook pp. 781-787)

1. Each year in the United States, approximately _____ million people have, or are at risk for developing, osteoporosis.

2. For osteoporosis to be visible on conventional radiographs, a loss of _____ % to _____ % of the trabecular bone must occur.

3. Cells responsible for new bone formation are called _____ , and cells that help to break

    down old bone are _____ .

4. Approximately at the age of _____ years, more bone is being removed than is being replaced by new bone formation.

5. The quantity or mass of bone measured in grams is the definition for _____ .

6. The purpose of bone densitometry is to:
   A. Establish the diagnosis of osteoporosis
   B. Assess the response to osteoporosis therapy
   C. Measure bone mineral density
   D. All of the above

7. Clinical indications for bone densitometry include all of the following *except:*
   A. Estrogen deficiency in women
   B. Hyperparathyrodism
   C. Vertebral abnormalities
   D. Polycystic kidney disease

8. True/False: Loss of magnesium and phosphorus from the bony cortex is the primary cause of osteoporosis

9. Place a check mark by each of the following that are *not* risk factors for osteoporosis as identified in the textbook:

   _____ A. Family history of osteoporosis

   _____ B. Excessive physical activity

   _____ C. Low sodium and niacin intake

   _____ D. Smoking

   _____ E. Low body weight

   _____ F. Alcohol consumption

   _____ G. High-fat diet

   _____ H. Low calcium intake

   _____ I. Height greater than 6 feet (180 cm)

   _____ J. Previous fractures

10. True/False: Women on estrogen replacement therapy (ERT) are at greater risk for acquiring osteoporotic fractures.

11. True/False: Bone strength and bone density are directly proportional.

12. True/False: Asian and Caucasian women have a greater risk for acquiring an osteoporotic fracture over other ethnic groups.

13. Osteoporosis in postmenopausal women is defined by the World Health Organization (WHO) as a bone mineral density (BMD) value of:

    A. 1.0 standard deviation below the average for the young normal population

    B. 1.5 standard deviations below the average for the same age and sex population

    C. 2.0 standard deviations below the average for the same age and sex population

    D. 2.5 standard deviations below the average for the young normal population

14. A T-score is defined as _____ .

15. A T-score of no lower than −1.0 indicates:

    A. Normal bone   C. Osteopenia

    B. Osteoporosis   D. Severe osteoporosis

16. Which of the following drugs given to treat or prevent osteoporosis is classified as a stimulator for new bone growth?

    A. Estrogen   C. Calcitonin

    B. Parathyroid hormone   D. Alendronate

17. True/False: Estrogen replacement therapy (ERT) is classified as an antiresorptive agent.

18. List the three most common diagnostic equivalent systems for bone densitometry:

    A. _____

    B. _____

    C. _____

19. Which of the following is the method of choice for evaluating both trabecular and cortical bone?

    A. Quantitative computed tomography (QCT)

    B. Dual-energy x-ray absorptiometry (DXA)

    C. Quantitative ultrasound (QUS)

    D. Dual-energy photon absorptiometry

20. What is the chief benefit of using a high and low x-ray energy source with a DXA system?

    A. Reduces patient dose significantly

    B. Reduces wear and tear on the x-ray tube

    C. Demonstrates attenuation differences between bone and soft tissue

    D. Reduces post-processing time of the digital image

21. Patient dose delivered during bone densitometry procedures using an x-ray source is measured in what units of

    measurement? _____

22. Average range of dose delivered during a DXA scan is _____ .

23. A Z-score produced during a DXA scan compares the patient's bone density with that of:

    A. An average young, healthy individual with peak bone mass

    B. An average individual of the same sex and age

    C. A person with a slight degree of osteoporosis

    D. A person with a severe degree of osteoporosis

24. QCT involves a scan taken between the vertebral levels of:

    A. C4 to T5

    B. T7 to T12

    C. T12 to L5

    D. L5 to S1

25. True/False: QCT permits three-dimensional analysis of the scanned region of the spine.

26. True/False: QCT produces less patient dose as compared with DXA.

27. Quantitative computed tomography (QCT) provides bone mineral density measurements of _____

    and _____ bone.

28. Average patient dose with QCT is approximately _____ .

29. The most common anatomic site selected for QUS is the :

    A. Spine   C. Os calcis

    B. Femur   D. Pelvis

30. Which of the following bone densitometry methods results in no radiation to the patient?

    A. DXA   C. QUS

    B. QCT   D. None of the above

31. Central or axial analysis using DXA or QCT includes bone density measurements of the:

    A. _____

    B. _____

32. True/False: Severe scoliosis or kyphosis may result in less accurate results for bone densitometry procedures.

33. True/False: If a patient had a previous fracture of the right hip, DXA should be performed on the right hip to gain a true measurement of BMD.

34. True/False: DXA of the hip requires the lower limb to be rotated 15° to 20° internally.

35. Another term for *precision* in regard to the ability of a DXA system to obtain repeated measurements on the same patient is:

    A. Reliability   C. Validity

    B. Reproducibility   D. Duplicity

36. Which of the following factors has the greatest impact of precision during a DXA scan?

    A. Patient positioning   C. Post-processing algorithm

    B. Exposure factors   D. Quality of x-ray beam

37. Typically, the accuracy of a DXA system is better than _____ %.

23

Laboratory Exercises

The following exercises involve two procedures for which supplies and equipment are most commonly available to students.

EXERCISE A: Orthoroentgenography-Long Bone Measurement (see textbook pp. 774-776)

1. Using an upper and lower limb radiographic phantom (if available), produce long bone measurement radiographs of the following:

    _____ Unilateral lower limb (AP projection of hip, knee, and ankle on one image receptor with a correctly placed Bell-Thompson ruler)

    _____ Bilateral lower limbs (AP projections of hips, knees, and ankles on one image receptor with correctly placed Bell-Thompson rulers)

    _____ Unilateral upper limb (AP projections of shoulder, elbow, and wrist on one image receptor with correctly placed ruler)

EXERCISE B: Conventional Tomography (see textbook pp. 777-780)

This part of the learning exercise needs to be carried out in an energized radiographic room equipped with a linear type tomographic unit. Check off the following steps as they are completed:

_____ **Step 1** **Equipment setup:** Set up the necessary tomographic equipment, including the adjustable fulcrum level attachment connected to the tube and to the Bucky. Ensure that the Bucky tray locks are released (as well as the tube angle and tube distance locks), allowing the tube and Bucky tray to move freely.

_____ **Step 2** **Preparation of "phantom" for experiments:** Design a series of experiments to demonstrate the tomographic blurring principle and the effect of the four controlling and influencing factors on blurring. Commercial tomographic phantoms are available with various lead numbers or other metallic devices placed at specific levels within the phantom. If these are not readily available, one can easily be made with paper clips in combination with a wire mesh or other flat metallic objects placed in horizontal layers in three different books or in three different layers within the same book. The shape or the configuration of the metallic objects can be varied in each layer so that the various levels can be differentiated on the radiograph.

_____ **Step 3** **Determine exposure factors:** Determine approximate exposure factors to visualize the metallic objects as placed in the books and stacked on the radiographic table. Start with an approximate upper limb exposure technique. Make a test exposure. Set the factors on the control panel of the tomographic unit as needed.

Optional Experiments to Demonstrate Tomographic Principles and Variables

Using your knowledge and understanding of tomographic blurring principles as studied in this chapter, design and carry out exercises as needed to demonstrate the following:

Experiment A: Orientation of Body Part to Tube Travel—Demonstrate that those objects parallel to the direction of tube movement create "streaks" and are not as effectively blurred as when they are perpendicular to the tube movement. This can be readily shown by changing the longitudinal direction of the metallic objects (e.g., paper clips) so that the levels above and below the focal plane will be at some angle or completely perpendicular to the direction of the tube travel. This should demonstrate increased blurring of the objects above and below the focal plane.

Experiment B: Influencing and Controlling Factors for Tomographic Blurring—Design experiments to demonstrate how each of the four factors or variables listed below influences or controls the amount of blurring. On these types of experiments, remember to change only one factor at a time, keeping all other factors constant.

_____ **Factor 1—Object-focal plane distance**

Demonstrate that those objects farther from the focal plane have greater movement on the image receptor and therefore increased blurring as compared with those closer to the focal plane.

This can be done by first taking tomographs with the objects above and below those in the focal plane. Compare these with tomographs taken when the objects above and below are placed at increased distances from the focal plane. You should be able to demonstrate markedly increased blurring on the second set of tomographs.

_____ **Factor 2—Exposure angle**

By changing the exposure angle, demonstrate that an increase in exposure angle with greater tube travel will increase the blurring, resulting in a thinner focal plane. Likewise, a decrease in exposure angle with less tube travel will decrease the movement of the objects above and below the focal plane, creating less blurring and a thicker section remaining in focus.

Remember that the amplitude or speed of tube movement must also increase as the exposure angle is increased so that the exposure continues throughout the full arc of tube travel.

_____ **Factor 3—Object image receptor distance (OID)**

Demonstrate that as the distance of the objects from the IR is increased, greater blurring will occur.

Sponge blocks can be placed between objects (e.g., books or phantom) and the table to increase the object-IR distance. (This will demonstrate why the upside or side away from the IR on a tomogram of a lateral TMJ or of a lateral of inner ear structures should be examined rather than the downside.)

Answers to Review Exercises

Review Exercise A: Arthrography

1. Synovial joints
2. Magnetic resonance imaging (MRI)
3. A. Tears of the joint capsule
   B. Tears of the menisci
   C. Tears of ligaments
4. Baker's cyst
5. Allergic reactions to iodine-based contrast media and allergic reactions to local anesthetics
6. True
7. False (needs to be flexed to distribute contrast media)
8. A. 10; 20; 5
   B. 50
9. A. Positive or radiopaque media such as iodinated, water-soluble contrast agent
   B. Negative or radiolucent contrast agents such as room air, oxygen, or carbon dioxide
10. A. AP
    B. Lateral
11. A. 20°
    B. 9
12. A. 6 views per meniscus
    B. 30°
13. A. Joint capsule
    B. Rotator cuff
    C. Long tendon of biceps muscle
    D. Articular cartilage
14. Rotator cuff
15. 2½- to 3½-inch spinal needle
16. A. 10 to 12 ml
    B. 3 to 4; 10 to 12
17. A. AP scout
    B. AP internal rotation
    C. AP external rotation
    D. Glenoid fossa (Grashey) projection
    E. Transaxillary (inferosuperior axial) projection
    F. Bicipital (intertubercular) groove projection
18. 15° to 23°

Review Exercise B: Hysterosalpingography

1. Uterus; uterine tubes
2. Rectosigmoid colon; urinary bladder
3. A. Fundus
   B. Corpus (or body)
   C. Isthmus
   D. Cervix
4. Corpus (or body)
5. Cervix
6. A. Endometrium
   B. Myometrium
   C. Serosa
7. A. Cornu
8. True
9. True
10. B. Patency
11. Assessment of female infertility
12. A. Demonstrate intrauterine pathology
    B. Evaluation of the uterine tubes following tubal ligation or reconstructive surgery
13. A. Endometrial polyps
    B. Uterine fibroids
    C. Intrauterine adhesions
14. A. Water-soluble, iodinated
15. Tenaculum
16. Slight Trendelenburg
17. A. LPO
    B. RPO
18. D. 2 inches (5 cm) superior to symphysis pubis

Review Exercise C: Myelography

1. A. Spinal cord
   B. Nerve root branches
2. A. Herniated nucleus pulposus (HNP)
   B. Cancerous or benign tumors
   C. Cysts
   D. Possible bone fragments
3. Herniated nucleus pulposus (HNP)
4. False (Most common are cervical and lumbar regions.)
5. A. Blood in the cerebrospinal fluid
   B. Arachnoiditis
   C. Increased intracranial pressure
   D. Recent lumbar puncture (within 2 weeks)
6. 90°/45° or 90°/90° tilting table
7. 1 hour
8. Subarachnoid space
9. A. Lumbar (L3-4)
   B. Cervical (C1-2)
10. Lumbar (L3-4)
11. A. Prone or left lateral
    B. Erect or prone
12. For spinal flexion to widen the interspinous spaces to facilitate needle placement
13. Nonionic, water-soluble, iodine-based
14. C. 1 hour
15. C. 6 to 17 ml
16. A. 4
    B. 5
    C. 8
    D. 1
    E. 6
    F. 2
    G. 7
    H. 3

17. Swimmer's lateral using a horizontal x-ray beam
18. To keep the contrast media from entering the cranial subarachnoid space
19. True (Right and left lateral decubitus positions are taken.)
20. 1. A. Horizontal beam lateral (prone), C5
       B. Horizontal beam lateral (swimmer's), C7
    2. A. R lateral decubitus (AP or PA), T7
       B. L lateral decubitus (AP or PA), T7
       C. R or L lateral, vertical beam, T7
    3. A. Semierect horizontal beam lateral (prone), L3
21. True

Review Exercise D: Sialography

1. A. Parotid glands
   B. Submandibular glands
   C. Sublingual glands
2. Parotid gland
3. Sublingual glands
4. A. Parotid duct
   B. Stensen's duct (older term)
5. D. Bartholin's duct
6. B. Ducts of Rivinus
7. Frenulum
8. A. Ducts of Rivinus
   B. Sublingual gland
   C. Submandibular duct (Wharton's duct)
   D. Parotid duct (Stensen's duct)
   E. Parotid gland
   F. Submandibular gland
9. A. Calculi
   B. Strictures
   C. Tumors
10. A. Dilation of the salivary duct
11. To cause the patient to produce saliva and help locate the opening of a particular duct
12. Lacrimal probe or a double-ended blunt
13. A. Butterfly needle
    B. Sialography catheter
14. Oil-based
15. Water-soluble
16. 1 to 2 ml
17. B. Sonography
18. A. Superoinferior projection

Review Exercise E: Orthoroentgenography

1. CT is more costly and requires specialized equipment.
2. A straight or right angle radiograph
3. To prevent elongation (magnification) of the limb as a result of the divergence of the x-ray beam
4. A special metallic (Bell-Thompson) ruler to measure bone length from one joint to another
5. Epiphysiodeses
6. Hip, knee, and ankle
7. True
8. True
9. A single center-placed ruler makes it difficult or impossible to shield the gonads without obscuring the upper part of the ruler.
10. True
11. False (PA would cross radius and ulna.)
12. False (The proximal humerus is rotated into an external rotation position.)

Review Exercise F: Conventional Tomography

1. A. The radiograph produced during a tomographic procedure
   B. The pivot point of the connecting rod between tube and IR
   C. The distance from table top to fulcrum
   D. The plane or section of the object that is clear and in focus
   E. The thickness of the objective plane
   F. The angle resulting from the x-ray tube beam movement
   G. The distance the tube travels
   H. The speed the tube travels in inches per second or cm per second
   I. The area of distortion of objects outside the objective plane
   J. The outer edges of the blurred object
2. Longitudinal and tube angle locks
3. False
4. False
5. A. Tube travel speed
   B. Objective plane
   C. Tube center
   D. Fulcrum level
6. False (Objects away from objective plane have greatest blurring.)
7. Objects farther from the fulcrum level or objective plane will be blurred by the movement of the tube and IR. Objects closer to this fulcrum level and those that are parallel to tube travel will remain almost stationary and experience little or no blurring.
8. A. Distance the object is from the objective plane
   B. Exposure angle
   C. Distance the object is from the IR (OID)
9. False (increases)
10. True
11. B. Perpendicular
12. C. 5°
13. D. 20°
14. True
15. Autotomography (or breathing technique)
16. Mandible studies
17. Slit beam restrictor or diaphragm

Review Exercise G: Bone Densitometry

1. 28
2. 30% to 50%
3. Osteoblasts; osteoclasts
4. 35 years
5. Bone mineral content (BMC)
6. D. All of the above
7. D. Polycystic kidney disease
8. False (loss of calcium and collagen)
9. B, C, G, I
10. False
11. True
12. True
13. D. 2.5 standard deviations below the average young normal population
14. The number of standard deviations an individual's BMD is from the mean BMD of an average, young individual of the same sex and ethnicity
15. A. Normal bone
16. B. Parathyroid hormone
17. True
18. A. Dual-energy x-ray absorptiometry (DXA)
    B. Quantitative computed tomography (QCT)
    C. Quantitative ultrasound (QUS)
19. A. Quantitative computed tomography (QCT)
20. C. Demonstrates attenuation differences between bone and soft tissue
21. MicroSeiverts (μSv)
22. 1 to 30 μSv
23. B. An average individual of the same sex and age
24. C. T12 to L5
25. True
26. False
27. Trabecular and cortical
28. 60 μSv
29. C. Os calcis
30. C. QUS
31. A. Lumbar spine
    B. Proximal femur
32. True
33. False
34. True
35. B. Reproducibility
36. A. Patient positioning
37. 10%

SELF-TEST

My Score = _____ %

This self-test should be taken only after completing all the readings, review exercises, and laboratory activities for a particular section. The purpose of this test is not only to provide a good learning exercise but also to serve as a good indicator of what your final evaluation exam will be. It is strongly suggested that if you do not get at least a 90% to 95% grade on this self-test, you review those areas in which you missed questions before going to your instructor for the final evaluation exam for this chapter. (There are 85 questions or blanks—each is worth 1.2 points.)

1. The formal term for a radiographic long bone measurement study is _____ .

2. True/False: To properly measure the length of a long bone, the entire lower limb should be included on a single projection.

3. True/False: Epiphysiodeses is an operation to lengthen bone by widening the epiphyseal plate.

4. True/False: Movement of the body part between exposures will compromise the long bone study.

5. True/False: If a long bone study of both lower limbs is ordered, the use of two metal rulers is recommended with both limbs exposed at the same time on the same image receptor.

6. What is the proper name for the special metal ruler used for long bone measurement? _____

7. What size of image receptor and how many exposures are recommended for a long bone study of the upper limbs

    for an adult (more than one answer possible)? _____

8. List the two synovial-type joints most commonly examined with an arthrogram.

    A. _____   B. _____

9. List the two contraindications for an arthrogram:

    A. _____   B. _____

10. An indication of a possible "Baker's cyst" would suggest the need for an arthrogram procedure for the _____ .

11. List the two types and the amounts of contrast media commonly used for a knee arthrogram:

	TYPE	*AMOUNT*
A.	_____	_____
B.	_____	_____

12. What size needle is most often used to introduce the contrast media during a knee arthrogram? _____

13. What is the purpose of flexing the knee gently after the contrast medium has been injected for an arthrogram procedure?

    _____

14. What size image receptor is recommended for horizontal beam arthrogram projections (more than one answer possible)?

    _____

15. How many exposures are made, and how much is the leg rotated, between each exposure for horizontal beam knee arthrograms?

    A. Number of exposures: _____

    B. Degrees of rotation between exposures: _____

16. The term *rotator cuff* refers to what structures of the shoulder? _____

17. What type of needle is most often used to introduce contrast media during a shoulder arthrogram? _____

18. List the overhead projections that may be requested for a shoulder arthrogram:

    Scout

    A. _____

    Postinjection

    B _____

    C. _____

    D. _____

    E. _____

    F. _____

19. List the four common lesions or conditions diagnosed through a myelogram:

    A. _____   C. _____

    B. _____   D. _____

20. List the four contraindications for a myelogram:

    A. _____   C. _____

    B. _____   D. _____

21. The most common clinical indication for a myelogram is:

    A. Benign tumors   C. HNP

    B. Spinal cysts   D. Bony injury to the spine

22. Where is the contrast medium injected during a myelogram? _____

23. Which position will move the contrast media column from the lumbar to the cervical region during a myelogram?

    A. Fowler's   C. Trendelenburg

    B. Left lateral decubitus   D. Prone

24. What is the most common spinal puncture site for a lumbar myelogram?

    A. L3-4   C. L4-5

    B. L1-2   D. L5 -S1

25. A cervical puncture is indicated for an upper spinal region myelogram if:

    A. The patient has severe lordosis   C. The patient has HNP of the L4-5 level

    B. The patient has mild scoliosis   D. The patient has complete blockage at T-spine level

26. The absorption of the water-soluble contrast media into the vascular system of the body begins approximately

    _____ minutes after injection and is totally undetectable radiographically after _____ hours.

27. Which position is performed during a cervical myelogram to demonstrate the C7-T1 region?

    _____

28. Another term for tomography is _____ .

29. Match each of the following tomographic terms with its correct definition:

    _____ A. Objective plane   1. The area of distortion

    _____ B. Exposure angle   2. The speed of tube travel

    _____ C. Tomogram   3. Radiograph produced by a tomographic unit

    _____ D. Blur   4. The plane where the object is clear

    _____ E. Fulcrum   5. The pivot point between tube and image receptor

    _____ F. Amplitude   6. The factor that determines slice thickness

30. True/False: Maximum blurring of an object will be achieved when it is perpendicular to tube travel.

31. True/False: The primary factor affecting the sectional thickness, as controlled by the operator, is amplitude.

32. True/False: Increased blurring occurs when the object is farther from the image receptor.

33. True/False: More blurring occurs with a shorter exposure angle.

34. True/False: In pantomography, the image receptor and tube move with the patient stationary similar to conventional tomography.

35. True/False: Amplitude does not influence or control the amount of blurring.

36. Which one of the following exposure times would be suitable for breathing technique (autotomography)?

    A. 2 to 3 seconds   C. ½ second

    B. 1 second   D. 10 milliseconds

37. List the four divisions of the uterus:

    A. _____   C. _____

    B. _____   D. _____

23

38. Which of the following is *not* a tissue layer of the uterus?

    A. Osseometrium   C. Endometrium

    B. Myometrium   D. Serosa

39. True/False: The uterine tubes are connected directly to the ovaries.

40. List the three contraindications for a hysterosalpingogram:

    A. _____

    B. _____

    C. _____

41. True/False: Oil-based contrast medium is preferred for the majority of hysterosalpingograms.

42. True/False: Hysterosalpingography can be a therapeutic tool in correcting certain obstructions in the uterine tube.

43. Match the following salivary ducts to the corresponding salivary gland:

    _____ A. Parotid gland   1. Ducts of Rivinus

    _____ B. Submandibular gland   2. Stensen's duct

    _____ C. Sublingual gland   3. Wharton's duct

44. Sialography is contraindicated for:

    A. Possible obstruction of the salivary duct   C. Salivary duct fistula

    B. Severe inflammation of the salivary gland or duct   D. Calculi lodged in salivary duct

45. What type of contrast media is more commonly used for sialograms?

    _____

46. What is the definition of sialectasia? _____

47. Which of the following is *not* a risk factor for osteoporosis?

    A. Excessive physical activity   C. Low body weight

    B. Alcohol consumption   D. Low calcium intake

48. Dual-energy x-ray absorptiometry (DXA) uses:

    A. Fan-beam x-ray source   C. Pencil-thin x-ray source

    B. Positron-emission source   D. Super voltage x-ray source

49. A T-score obtained with the DXA system compares the patient with a(n):

    A. Average patient of the same age, sex, and ethnic background

    B. Young healthy individual with peak bone mass

    C. Young healthy individual of the same sex and ethnic background

    D. Patient with severe osteoporosis

50. The two disadvantages of quantitative computed tomography (QCT) are:

    A. _____

    B. _____

51. The anatomic area most commonly scanned with quantitative ultrasound (QUS) is the _____ .

52. What specific cells are responsible for bone resorption? _____

53. Which of the following factors often leads to advanced bone loss?

    A. Being a female over the age of 21 years   C. Undergoing glucocorticoid therapy

    B. Undergoing hormone replacement therapy   D. Undergoing cardiac rehab

54. True/False: African-American women are at greater risk for developing osteoporosis than are Caucasian women.

55. A T-score acquired during a DXA scan of lower than −1.0 but higher than −2.5 indicates:

    A. Normal BMD   C. Osteoporosis

    B. Osteopenia   D. Severe osteoporosis

56. True/False: Estrogen replacement therapy (ERT) stimulates new bone formation.

57. What is the range of dose delivered to a patient during a DXA scan?

    A. 1 to 30 μSv   C. 1 to 30 Seiverts

    B. 40 to 60 μSv   D. 1 to 3 mSv

58. True/False: As the technology is refined, QUS may replace existing peripheral techniques.

59. Which vertebral region(s) is(are) analyzed during a DXA scan?

    A. T12   C. L1 to L4

    B. Between T7 and L1   D. L4 to S1

60. The ability of a DXA system to obtain consistent BMD values of repeated measurements of the same patient is

    called _____ .

CHAPTER 24

Additional Diagnostic and Therapeutic Modalities

This chapter introduces select alternative diagnostic and therapeutic imaging modalities, including **nuclear medicine (NM)**, **positron emission tomography (PET)**, **radiation oncology (therapy)**, **diagnostic ultrasound (sonography)**, and **magnetic resonance imaging (MRI)**. The information and review exercises contained in Chapter 24 are intended to introduce students to basic concepts related to each of these modalities. Basic definitions, physical principles, clinical applications, and technologist responsibilities will be covered.

A more extensive presentation is provided in the MRI section, which introduces MRI terminology and the basics of MRI physics and instrumentation. The important clinical aspects related to personnel and patient safety are discussed. An introduction to the imaging parameters that affect the quality of the images and clinical applications of MRI is included.

CHAPTER OBJECTIVES

After you have successfully completed all the activities of this chapter, you will be able to:

_____ 1. Identify basic operating principles related to nuclear medicine imaging.

_____ 2. List the purpose, radionuclide used, and pathologic indications demonstrated with select nuclear medicine procedures.

_____ 3. List specific responsibilities for members of the nuclear medicine team.

_____ 4. Describe the PET imaging process.

_____ 5. Identify the different types of radionuclides used in PET imaging.

_____ 6. Describe the basic operating principles of PET imaging.

_____ 7. Identify the pathologic conditions best demonstrated with PET imaging.

_____ 8. Define terms and concepts specific to nuclear medicine technology.

_____ 9. Distinguish between internal and external types of radiation therapy.

_____ 10. Identify the energy level, characteristics, and advantages of the major types of radiation therapy units.

_____ 11. List the specific responsibilities of radiation oncology team members.

_____ 12. Identify basic operating principles related to ultrasound.

_____ 13. List the characteristics, advantages, and disadvantages of specific types of ultrasound systems.

_____ 14. List the purpose, transducer used, and pathologic indications demonstrated with select ultrasound procedures.

_____ 15. Explain how MRI produces an image.

_____ 16. Compare the process of MRI image production with that of other imaging modalities.

_____ 17. Explain how a tissue signal is generated and received from body tissues.

_____ 18. Explain how image contrast is produced in the MR image.

_____ 19. Identify basic MRI safety considerations.

_____ 20. Identify information to be included when preparing a patient for an MRI exam.

_____ 21.   Identify the type of contrast agent used in MRI.

_____ 22.   State the appearance of specific tissue types on both T1- and T2-weighted images.

_____ 23.   Define the terms and pathologic indications related to MRI.

_____ 24.   Explain the purpose and applications of functional MRI (fMRI).

Learning Exercises

The following review exercises should be completed only after careful study of the associated pages in the textbook, as indicated by each exercise. Answers to each review exercise are given at the end of the review exercises.

REVIEW EXERCISE A: Nuclear Medicine and PET (see textbook pp. 786-791)

1.   Nuclear medicine uses radioactive materials called _____ in the study and treatment of various medical conditions.

2.   Radioactive materials that are introduced into the body and concentrate in specific organs are called

_____ .

3.   How are the materials identified in question 2 introduced into the body?

A.   Inhalation   C.   Injection

B.   Orally   D.   All of the above

4.   One of the most common radioactive materials used in nuclear medicine procedures is:

A.   Sulfur colloid   C.   Technetium 99m

B.   Iodine 131   D.   Thallium

5.   *SPECT* is an abbreviation for: _____ .

6.   The SPECT camera provides a _____ -dimensional view of the anatomy.

7.   A study of the skeletal system using radioactive materials is called _____ .

8.   A common genitourinary nuclear medicine study is performed for:

A.   Kidney transplants   C.   Pyelonephritis

B.   Renal cyst   D.   All of the above

9.   Nuclear medicine is considered the ideal modality for diagnosing _____ of the gastrointestinal tract.

A.   Peptic ulcers   C.   Gastroesophageal reflux

B.   Meckel's diverticulum   D.   Colitis

10.   Which one of the following radiopharmaceuticals is used during myocardial perfusion studies?

A.   Technetium 99m   C.   Iodine 131

B.   Thallium   D.   Neo Tect

11.   Which one of the following radiopharmaceuticals is used to determine whether a pulmonary lesion is benign or malignant?

A.   Technetium 99m   C.   Iodine 131

B.   Thallium   D.   Neo Tect

12. Match the following responsibilities to the correct nuclear medicine team member:

_____ A. Properly disposes of contaminated materials   1. Nuclear medicine technologist

_____ B. Calibrates nuclear medicine imaging equipment   2. Nuclear medicine physician

_____ C. Performs statistical analysis of study data   3. Medical nuclear physicist

_____ D. Administers radionuclide to patient

_____ E. Interprets procedure

_____ F. Often serves as department radiation safety officer

_____ G. Licensed to acquire and use radioactive materials

_____ H. Prepares radioactive materials

_____ I. Digitally processes the images

13. Match each of the following nuclear medicine terms to its correct definition (use each choice only once):

_____ A. Synonym for a product of decay   1. Becquerel

_____ B. Time required for disintegration of original energy   2. Radionuclide half of a radioactive nuclei

     3. Daughter

_____ C. Type of atom whose nucleus disintegrates spontaneously   4. Curie

_____ D. Test substance labeled with a marker such as a radioactive isotope or a fluorescent compound   5. Equilibrium

     6. Half-life

_____ E. SI unit of radioactivity   7. Disintegration

_____ F. Stage in a reaction where the concentration of the reactive species is no longer changing   8. Tracer

_____ G. Traditional or standard unit of radioactivity

_____ H. Spontaneous nuclear transformation characterized by the emission of energy and/or mass from the nucleus

14. *PET* is an acronym for: _____ .

15. PET is a process that demonstrates:

A. Anatomic appearance of tissues and organs

B. Molecular make-up of tissues

C. Biochemical function of the body's organs and tissue

D. Pathologic processes of brain tissue only

16. True/False: The PET scanner produces radiation with an intensity of 5.11 keV.

17. PET uses radioactive compounds that emit _____ during the radioactive decay process.

    A. Electrons   C. Two gamma rays

    B. Positrons   D. Neutrinos

18. The PET scanner detector array measures:

    A. Emitted photons   C. Positrons

    B. Electrons   D. Neutrons

19. PET uses radioactive compounds, which include oxygen and nitrogen, as well as:

    A. Selenium and iron   C. Carbon and argon

    B. Hydrogen and iodine   D. Carbon and fluorine

20. PET radioactive compounds measure all of the following vital cellular processes *except:*

    A. Oxygen utilization   C. Cellular reproduction

    B. Tissue perfusion   D. Glucose metabolism

21. Match each of the following PET tracer compounds to the cellular function that it measures (different compounds may measure the same biologic process):

    _____ A. Glucose metabolism   1. ^{13}N-ammonia

    _____ B. Blood flow/perfusion   2. ^{18}F-FDG

    _____ C. Amino acid metabolism   3. ^{15}O-water

                                           4. ^{11}C-methionine

22. What is the name of the device required to produce the PET radioactive compounds? _____

23. Most PET tracers have a half-life of:

    A. 120 seconds to 110 minutes   C. 15 minutes to 8 hours

    B. 10 to 60 seconds   D. 8 to 12 hours

24. True/False: PET is superior to MRI in demonstrating anatomic structures of the brain.

25. True/False: Often PET can detect abnormal function of the brain prior to the onset of actual symptoms.

26. PET is most often used in the areas of neurology, cardiology, and:

    A. Urology   C. Orthopedics

    B. Endocrinology   D. Oncology

27. PET plays an important role in the initial diagnosis and _____ of malignancy.

    A. Destruction   C. Staging

    B. Prevention   D. Cure

28. True/False: Active tumor growth will lead to a decreased uptake of FDG.

29. True/False: Decreased uptake of an ammonia tracer in the heart tissue may indicate that coronary artery disease (CAD) is present.

30. PET is used in the study of epileptic patients to:

    A. Identify seizure locations in the brain

    B. Minimize the recurrence of seizures

    C. Examine the white matter of the brain

    D. Calculate the rate or frequency of seizures

31. PET brain mapping is performed to:

    A. Identify possible tumors in the brain

    B. Distinguish between the gray and white matter of the brain

    C. Identify the transmission or impulse patterns of the brain

    D. Identify the location of key motor and sensory regions of the brain

32. In patients with Alzheimer's disease, glucose metabolism is dramatically _____ (**increased**

    or **decreased**) in several key areas of the brain.

33. Coregistration is another term for:

    A. PET image manipulation

    B. Increased tracer uptake in the brain

    C. Artifact seen on certain PET image

    D. Fusion technology

34. PET may be combined with _____ to produce both an anatomic and functional evaluation

    of the anatomy.

35. True/False: It is possible to acquire functional PET and anatomic CT images in the same scanning session when the correct technology is employed.

REVIEW EXERCISE B: Radiation Oncology (Therapy) (see textbook p. 792)

1. Cancer is second only to _____ as the leading cause of death in the United States and Canada.

2. Identify the two types of radiation therapy treatment:

    A. _____

    B. _____

3. Prostate cancer is a common candidate for which of the two types of radiation therapy treatment from question 2?

    _____

4. List the three sources of external beam radiation:

    A. _____

    B. _____

    C. _____

5. Cobalt-60 units emit gamma rays at the intensity of _____ MeV.

    A. 1.25   C. 10.4

    B. 5.25   D. 15.25

6. What is the source of the high-energy x-rays produced with a linear accelerator therapy unit?

    A. Cobalt-60   C. Uranium 235

    B. High-speed neutrons striking an anode   D. High-speed electrons striking an anode

7. Which of the following is most effective for the treatment of shallow or superficial cancerous tissue?

    A. Cobalt-60   C. High-voltage x-ray type unit

    B. Linear accelerator   D. Internal, brachytherapy type

8. Linear accelerators produce energy levels between _____ MeV.

    A. 1 to 2   C. 4 to 30

    B. 3 to 5   D. 30 to 50

9. What is the purpose of radiation therapy simulation? _____

10. Match the following responsibilities to the correct radiation oncology team member:

    _____ A. Outlines plan to deliver the desired dosage   1. Radiation therapist

    _____ B. Administers radiation treatments   2. Radiation oncologist

    _____ C. May use fluoroscopy to determine treatment fields   3. Medical dosimetrist

    _____ D. Calibrates equipment   4. Medical health physicist

    _____ E. Prescribes treatment plan

    _____ F. Advises oncologists on dosage calculations

    _____ G. Maintains treatment records

REVIEW EXERCISE C: Ultrasound (see textbook pp. 793-796)

1. List three additional terms for ultrasound:

    A. _____

    B. _____

    C. _____

2. Medical ultrasound uses high-frequency sound waves in the range between _____ to _____ MHz.

3. True/False: Ultrasound is an ideal imaging modality for diagnosing an ileus.

4. True/False: Ultrasound is often used to locate a bone cyst in the femur.

5. True/False: Research studies conclude that there are no adverse biologic effects associated with the use of medical ultrasound.

6. True/False: The first A-mode ultrasound unit was built in Germany in the late 1960s.

7. Which generation of ultrasound unit introduced two-dimensional gray scale?

    A. A-mode   C. Real-time dynamic

    B. B-mode   D. Doppler

8. Which type of ultrasound unit is used to examine the structure and behavior of flowing blood?

    A. A-mode   C. Real-time dynamic

    B. B-mode   D. Doppler

9. What major improvement is offered by the new high-definition digital ultrasound systems?

    A. Smaller size unit   C. Increase in dynamic range

    B. Can alter between A-mode and B-mode   D. Introduction of gray scale

10. What is the fundamental purpose or function of the transducer? _____

11. What type of material comprises the functional aspect of the transducer, which creates the high-frequency sound waves?

    A. Tungsten alloy   C. Silver/chromium alloy

    B. Ceramic   D. Ferrous alloy

12. What physical principle is applied when the transducer produces a sound wave?

    A. Piezoelectric effect   C. Thermionic emission

    B. Modulation transfer   D. Larmor effect

13. Match the following procedures and/or situations to the correct frequency transducer (use each choice only once):

    _____   A. For an average or small abdomen   1. 3.5 MHz

    _____   B. For a larger abdomen   2. 5.0 to 7.0 MHz

    _____   C. For a study of a superficial structure   3. 17 MHz

14. True/False: A transducer serves as both a transmitter and receiver of echoes.

15. True/False: A sonographer must provide initial interpretation of the ultrasound images.

16. Ultrasound is the "gold standard" for studies of all of the following structures *except* the:

    A. Liver   C. Gallbladder

    B. Stomach   D. Uterus

17. What is the name of the ultrasound procedure in which amniotic fluid is withdrawn from the uterus for genetic analysis?

    _____

18. Ultrasound is very effective in evaluating the fetus before birth for early indications of:

    A. Heart defects   C. Spina bifida

    B. Hydrocephaly   D. All of the above

19. What is the advantage of using ultrasound instead of MRI for studies of the musculoskeletal system?

    A. Less expensive   C. Provides a functional study of joint movement

    B. Noninvasive   D. All of the above

¹/20 of these

20. Match each of the following sonographic terms to its correct definition (use each choice only once):

    _____ A. An image that possesses both width and height

    _____ B. Alteration in frequency or wavelength reflected by movement

    _____ C. Acoustic energy that travels through a medium

    _____ D. An anatomic object that does not produce any echoes

    _____ E. Ultrasound images that demonstrate dynamic motion

    _____ F. An anatomic object that produces more echoes than normal

    _____ G. Acoustic energy reflected from a structure that interferes

    _____ H. An anatomic structure that possesses echo-producing structures

    _____ I. An aspect of acoustic energy reflected back toward the source or origin

    _____ J. An anatomic object that produces fewer echoes than normal

1. Anechoic
2. Backscatter objects
3. Doppler effect
4. Echogenic
5. Hyperechoic
6. Hypoechoic
7. Real-time imaging with the expected path of the acoustic wave
8. Two-dimensional image
9. Wave
10. Reflection

REVIEW EXERCISE D: Physical Principles of MRI (see textbook pp. 797-801)

1. MRI uses _____ and _____ to obtain a mathematically reconstructed image.

2. The MRI image represents differences in the patient's tissues in the number of _____ and the rate at which they recover from radiofrequency stimulation.

3. To compare the energy of x-rays and MRI radio waves and the relative effect on irradiated tissue, fill in the blanks in the following:

		WAVELENGTH	*FREQUENCY*	*ENERGY*
1.	Typical x-rays	A. 10^{-11} M	B. 10^{19} Hz cycles/sec	C. 60,000 electron volts
2.	MRI radio waves	A. _____	B. _____	C. _____

4. A. Which nucleus is most suitable for MRI? _____

    B. Why? _____

5. Which component of the nucleus is affected by radio waves and static magnetic fields? _____

6. A typical cubic centimeter of the human body may contain approximately how many hydrogen atoms?

    A. 1022   C. 10^{10}

    B. 10,020   D. 10^{20}

7. Define *precession* by comparing it to another, more well-known phenomenon.

    _____

8. The rate of precession of a proton in a magnetic field _____ (**increases** or **decreases**) as the strength of the magnetic field increases.

9. Precession occurs as a result of _____ acting on a spinning nuclei.

10. The angle of precession of protons can be altered by the introduction of _____ .

11. How does an increase in the length of application time of the radio wave affect the angle of precession of the exposed nuclei?

    _____

12. Timing of the radio wave frequency to the rate of the precessing nuclei is an example of the concept of

    _____ .

13. The signal that is received by the antenna or the receiving coil comes from which part of the atoms in the body tissues?

    _____

14. The nucleus emits _____ waves because it is a tiny magnet that is also

    _____ .

15. Relaxation of the nuclei as soon as the radiofrequency pulse is turned off can be divided into two categories:

    _____ and _____ .

16. T1 relaxation is known as _____ (**transverse** or **longitudinal**), or spin-lattice, relaxation.

17. T2 relaxation is known as _____ (**transverse** or **longitudinal**), or spin-spin, relaxation.

18. The quantity of hydrogen nuclei per given volume of tissue is referred to as the _____ ,

    which is a _____ (**major** or **minor**) contributor to the appearance of the MR image.

19. Describe the main purpose of the gradient magnetic fields (the magnetic field strengths through only specific regions or slices of body tissue).

    _____

20. What are three primary factors that determine the signal strength and therefore the brightness of an image?

    A. _____

    B. _____

    C. _____

24

REVIEW EXERCISE E: Clinical Applications, Safety Considerations, and Appearance of Anatomy (see textbook pp. 803-806)

1. Complete the following list of MRI safety concerns:

    A. _____

    B. _____

    C. _____

    D. Local heating of tissues and metallic objects

    E. Electrical interference with normal functions of nerve cells and muscle fibers

2. The danger of projectiles becomes _____ (**greater** or **lesser**) as ferromagnetic objects are

    moved toward the scanner because the field strength is _____ (**directly** or **inversely**) proportional to the cube of the distance from the bore of the magnet.

3. In a code blue (emergency) situation, the patient is removed from the scan room because of the danger of

    _____ .

4. Pacemakers are not allowed inside the _____ -gauss line.

5. As a general rule, O_2 tanks, IV pumps, and wheelchairs are not allowed inside the _____ -gauss line.

6. Magnetic tapes, credit cards, and cochlear implants are not allowed inside the _____ -gauss line.

7. The most important contraindication to MRI of the brain involves torquing of _____ .

8. What unit of measurement is used to calculate local heating of tissues? (HINT: Initials are SAR.)

    _____

9. MRI has the ability to demonstrate anatomy in _____ , _____ , and

    _____ planes.

10. MRI has excellent _____ , which allows visualization of soft-tissue structures.

11. Diagnosis of diseases such as those involving the CNS can be made with MRI by comparing the signals produced

    in _____ (**normal** or **abnormal**) tissues with those produced in

    _____ (**normal** or **abnormal**) tissues.

12. List three types of histories that should be obtained from patients before an MRI exam.

   A. _____   C. _____

   B. _____

13. Name the IV contrast agent most commonly used in MRI: _____

14. Describe how the contrast agent identified in question 13 affects T1 and T2 relaxation rates: _____

   _____

15. The average amount of contrast media given during an MRI examination is _____ ml/kg; the injection rate

   should not exceed _____ ml/min.

16. List eight absolute contraindications to patient MRI scanning as listed in the textbook.

   A. _____

   B. _____

   C. _____

   D. _____

   E. _____

   F. _____

   G. _____

   H. _____

17. Match the following pulse sequence descriptions with the correct designation.

   _____ A. Pulse sequences using a combination of short TR and short TE   1. T1 relaxation

   _____ B. Pulse sequences using a combination of long TR and long TE   2. T2 relaxation

18. For each tissue listed below, identify the T1- and T2-weighted appearances: dark, bright, light gray, or dark gray
   (NOTE: The first tissue has been completed as an example):

		T1	*T2*
A.	Cortical bone	Dark	Dark
B.	Red bone marrow	_____	_____
C.	Fat	_____	_____
D.	White brain matter	_____	_____
E.	CSF	_____	_____
F.	Muscle	_____	_____
G.	Vessels	_____	_____

19. True/False: Flowing blood is not visualized with a conventional spin-echo pulse sequence.

20. True/False: Tissues filled with air do not produce a T1 or T2 signal and therefore appear as bright.

REVIEW EXERCISE F: MRI Examinations (see textbook: pp. 807-809)

1. Complete the list of six structures or tissue types best demonstrated by MRI of the brain:

    A. Gray matter   D. _____

    B. _____   E. Basal ganglia

    C. _____   F. Brain stem

2. Complete the list of six possible pathologies demonstrated by MRI of the brain:

    A. _____   D. _____

    B. _____   E. Hemorrhagic disorders

    C. _____   F. CVA

3. MRI of the brain is considered superior to the CT in visualizing the following three regions of the brain or changes in tissues:

    A. _____

    B. _____

    C. _____

4. Which of the following technical factors may be used in spine imaging?
    A. T1-weighted sequence   C. Cardiac gating
    B. T2-weighted sequence   D. All of the above

5. MRI of the spine is effective in evaluating:

    A. _____

    B. _____

    C. _____

6. List two major advantages of MRI over CT imaging of the spine.

    A. _____

    B. _____

7. True/False: CT is superior to MRI for evaluation of spinal trauma.

8. List the four conditions or diseases best demonstrated with MRI of the joints:

A. _____

B. _____

C. _____

D. _____

9. MRI of the abdomen is helpful in identifying tumors containing _____ .

10. True/False: Sonography and CT are the modalities of choice for demonstrating renal cysts.

11. True/False: As magnet or field strength increases, quality and resolution of the MR image increase.

12. True/False: Cardiac gating during an MRI procedure is a process in which heart wall motion is studied.

13. True/False: During the cardiac-gated MRI procedure, signal collection occurs at the same point during the cardiac cycle.

14. Which one of the following devices/equipment is required during a cardiac-gated MRI procedure?

A. CT   C. PET

B. ECG   D. Pulse oximeter

15. True/False: Functional MRI (fMRI) provides both an anatomic and functional assessment of the brain.

16. Neural activity is measured by _____ during a functional MRI procedure.

A. Decreased RF signal   C. Blood oxygen level dependent (BOLD) signal

B. Increased RF signal   D. Water shift signal

17. True/False: fMRI does not require the injection of radiopharmaceuticals.

18. True/False: fMRI scan times are typically longer than similar PET studies of the brain.

19. True/False: Spatial image resolution with fMRI is less than with PET or SPECT.

20. Match the following MRI terms with the correct definition (refer to textbook p. 810 for questions 20 and 21):

_____ A. MRI technique to minimize involuntary motion artifacts   1. T2

_____ B. False features on an image caused by patient instability or   2. Tesla
            equipment deficiencies
                                                                               3. Signal averaging
_____ C. Slow gyration of an axis of a spinning body caused by an
            application of torque   4. Acoustic neuroma

_____ D. Method of improving SNR by averaging several FIDs or spin echoes   5. Fringe field

_____ E. Spin lattice or longitudinal relaxation time   6. Schwannoma

_____ F. SI unit of magnetic field intensity   7. Artifacts

_____ G. Stray magnetic field that exists outside the imager   8. Physiologic gating

_____ H. A new growth of the white substance of the nerve sheath   9. Precession

_____ I. A tumor growing from nerve cells affecting the sense of hearing   10. T1

_____ J. Spin-spin or transverse relaxation time

21.   Match the following MRI terms with the correct definition:

_____   A.   Measure of the geometric relationship between the RF coil and the body   1.   Contrast resolution

_____   B.   Atmospheric gases such as nitrogen and helium used for cooling   2.   Chordoma

_____   C.   Reappearance of MR signal after the FID has disappeared   3.   Turbulence

_____   D.   Amount of rotation of the net magnetization vector produced by an RF puls   4.   Spin echo

_____   E.   Force that causes or tends to cause a body to rotate   5.   Filling factor

_____   F.   Repetition time   6.   Meningioma

_____   G.   In flowing fluid, velocity component that fluctuates randomly   7.   Cryogen

_____   H.   A malignant tumor arising from the embryonic remains of the notocord   8.   Torque

_____   I.   A hard, slow-growing vascular tumor   9.   TR

_____   J.   Ability of an imaging process to distinguish adjacent soft-tissue   10.   Flip angle
                structures from one another

Answers to Review Exercises

Review Exercise A: Nuclear Medicine and PET

1. Radiopharmaceuticals
2. Tracers
3. D. All of the above
4. C. Technetium 99m
5. Single photon emission computed tomography
6. Three
7. Bone scintigraphy
8. A. Kidney transplants
9. B. Meckel's diverticulum
10. B. Thallium
11. D. Neo Tect
12. A. 1
    B. 3
    C. 1
    D. 1
    E. 2
    F. 3
    G. 2
    H. 3
    I. 1
13. A. 3
    B. 6
    C. 2
    D. 8
    E. 1
    F. 5
    G. 4
    H. 7
14. Positron emission tomography
15. C. Biochemical function of the body's organs and tissue
16. False (The PET scanner itself does not produce radiation.)
17. B. Positrons
18. A. Emitted photons
19. D. Carbon and fluorine
20. C. Cellular reproduction
21. A. 2
    B. 1, 2, 3
    C. 4
22. Cyclotron
23. A. 120 seconds to 110 minutes
24. False
25. True
26. D. Oncology
27. C. Staging
28. False
29. True
30. A. Identify seizure locations in the brain
31. D. Identify the location of key motor and sensory regions of the brain
32. Decreased
33. D. Fusion technology
34. MRI or CT
35. True

Review Exercise B: Radiation Oncology (Therapy)

1. Heart-related diseases
2. A. Internal, brachytherapy
    B. External beam, teletherapy
3. Internal, brachytherapy
4. A. X-ray units
    B. Cobalt-60 gamma rays units
    C. Linear accelerator or betatron units
5. A. 1.25
6. D. High-speed electrons striking an anode
7. B. Linear accelerator
8. C. 4 to 30
9. To determine the area and volume of tissue to be treated
10. A. 3
    B. 1
    C. 1
    D. 4
    E. 2
    F. 4
    G. 1

Review Exercise C: Ultrasound

1. A. Sonography
    B. Ultrasonography
    C. Echosonography
2. 1 to 17
3. False (not ideal for ileus)
4. False (not used for bone cyst)
5. True
6. False (in the early 1950s)
7. B. B-mode
8. D. Doppler
9. C. Increase in dynamic range
10. Converts electrical energy to ultrasonic energy
11. B. Ceramic
12. A. Piezoelectric effect
13. A. 2
    B. 1
    C. 3
14. True
15. True
16. B. Stomach
17. Amniocentesis
18. D. All of the above
19. D. All of the above
20. A. 8
    B. 3
    C. 9
    D. 1
    E. 7
    F. 5
    G. 10
    H. 4
    I. 2
    J. 6

Review Exercise D: Physical Principles of MRI

1. Magnetic fields and radio waves
2. Nuclei
3. 2. A. 10^3 to 10^{-2} meters
    B. 10^5 to 10^{10} hertz
    C. 10^{-7} electron volts (eV)
4. A. Hydrogen (single-proton nucleus)
    B. The large amount of hydrogen present in any organism
5. Proton
6. A. 1022
7. Is similar to the wobble of a slowly spinning top
8. Increases
9. An outside force (the magnetic field)
10. Radio waves
11. Increase in time increases the angle of precession
12. Resonance
13. Nucleus or proton
14. Radio; precessing or rotating
15. T1 relaxation and T2 relaxation
16. Longitudinal
17. Transverse
18. Spin density; minor
19. So that the returning signal can be located (because only the precessing nuclei within these regions or slice transmit signals).
20. A. Spin density
    B. T1 relaxation rate
    C. T2 relaxation rate

Review Exercise E: Clinical Applications, Safety Considerations, and Appearance of Anatomy

1. A. Potential hazards of projectiles
    B. Electrical interference with implants
    C. Torquing of ferromagnetic objects
2. Greater; directly
3. Danger of ferromagnetic objects used in code blue (emergency) situations becoming projectiles
4. 5
5. 50
6. 10
7. Ferromagnetic intracranial aneurysm clips
8. Specific absorption ratio
9. Transverse, sagittal, and coronal
10. Contrast resolution
11. Normal; abnormal
12. A. Surgical history
    B. Occupational history
    C. Accidental history

13. Gd-DTPA (gadolinium-DTPA)
14. Shortens T1 and T2 relaxation rates
15. 0.2; 10
16. A. Cardiac pacemakers
    B. Electronic implant
    C. Ferromagnetic aneurysm clip in the brain
    D. Inner ear surgery
    E. Metallic fragments in the body
    F. Metal in and/or removed from the eye
    G. Eye prostheses
    H. Pregnancy
17. A. 1
    B. 2

18.

	T1	T2
B.	Light gray	Dark gray
C.	Bright	Dark
D.	Light gray	Dark gray
E.	Dark	Bright
F.	Dark gray	Dark gray
G.	Dark	Dark

19. True
20. False (appear black)

Review Exercise F: MRI Examinations

1. B. White matter
   C. Nerve tissue
   D. Ventricles

2. A. White matter disease (multiple sclerosis or demyelinating disease)
   B. Ischemic disorders
   C. Neoplasm
   D. Infectious diseases (such as AIDS and herpes)
3. A. Posterior fossa
   B. Brain stem
   C. Detecting small changes in tissue water content
4. D. All of the above
5. A. Cysts
   B. Syrinx
   C. Lipomas
6. A. MRI does not require the use of intrathecal ("within a sheath") contrast media.
   B. MRI covers a large area of the spine in a single sagittal view.
7. True
8. A. Soft-tissue tumors
   B. Osteonecrosis
   C. Ligament tears
   D. Tendon tears
9. Fat
10. True
11. True
12. False

13. True
14. B. ECG
15. True
16. C. Blood oxygen level dependent (BOLD) signal
17. True
18. False
19. False
20. A. 8
    B. 7
    C. 9
    D. 3
    E. 10
    F. 2
    G. 5
    H. 6
    I. 4
    J. 1
21. A. 5
    B. 7
    C. 4
    D. 10
    E. 8
    F. 9
    G. 3
    H. 2
    I. 6
    J. 1

SELF-TEST

My Score = _____ %

This self-test should be taken only after completing all of the readings, review exercises, and laboratory activities for a particular section. The purpose of this test is not only to provide a good learning exercise but also to serve as a good indicator of what your final evaluation exam will be. It is strongly suggested that if you do not get at least a 90% to 95% grade on this self-test, you review those areas where you missed questions before going to your instructor for the final evaluation exam for this chapter. (There are 85 questions or blanks—each is worth 1.3 points.)

1. One of the most common radionuclides used in nuclear medicine is:

    A. Thallium   C. Cardiolyte

    B. Technetium 99m   D. Sulfur colloid

2. What type of imaging device used in nuclear medicine provides a three-dimensional image of anatomic structures?

    A. SPECT camera   C. Linear accelerator

    B. B-mode unit   D. Real-time scanner

3. An abnormal region detected during a nuclear medicine skeletal scan is often described as a(n):

    A. Signal void   C. Acoustic shadow

    B. Hot spot   D. Region of high attenuation

4. Which one of the following is a common pathologic indicator for a nuclear medicine gastrointestinal study?

    A. Duodenal ulcer   C. Meckel's diverticulum

    B. Bezoar   D. Ileus

5. If a treadmill is not available for a nuclear medicine cardiac study, the patient is given:

    A. Glucagon   C. Lasix

    B. Valium   D. Vasodilator

6. True/False: The perfusion phase of a nuclear medicine lung ventilation/perfusion study is performed **before** the ventilation phase.

7. Which one of the following duties is *not* a typical responsibility of the nuclear medicine technologist?

    A. Calibrates instrumentation   C. Administers radionuclides

    B. Process images   D. Decontaminates area after spills

8. Which one of the following is *not* an example of a teletherapy unit?

    A. Linear accelerator   C. X-ray units

    B. Neutron accelerator   D. Cobalt-60 unit

9. Linear accelerators deliver energy levels to target tissues between:

    A. 50 to 100 kV   C. 100 to 300 kV

    B. 1.25 to 5.0 MeV   D. 4 to 30 MeV

10. True/False: The patient is often skin-tattooed during radiation therapy simulations.

24

11. Which one of the following is *not* a responsibility of the certified radiation therapist?

    A. Uses fluoroscopy for treatment planning   C. Prescribes the treatment

    B. Interacts directly with the patient   D. Maintains therapy records

12. Which of the following is *not* an alternative term for medical ultrasound?

    A. Echosonography   C. Piezosonography

    B. Sonography   D. Ultrasonography

13. Medical ultrasound operates at a frequency range between:

    A. 1 to 5 KHz   C. 1 to 17 KHz

    B. 25 to 50 KHz   D. 1 to 17 MHz

14. Which generation of ultrasound equipment first introduced gray scale imaging?

    A. A-mode   C. Real-time dynamic

    B. B-mode   D. Doppler

15. An ultrasound transducer converts _____ energy to ultrasonic energy.

    A. Electrical   C. Light

    B. Heat   D. Magnetic

16. Which of the following transducer frequencies would most likely be used on a large abdomen?

    A. 3.5 MHz   C. 10 MHz

    B. 5.0 to 7.0 MHz   D. 17 MHz

17. True/False: A higher-frequency transducer will increase penetration through the anatomy but will produce lower image resolution.

18. True/False: A normal gallbladder is an example of a *hyperechoic* structure.

19. True/False: Breast ultrasound is used primarily to distinguish between solid and cystic masses.

20. With color-flow Doppler, blood flowing away from the transducer is:

    A. Red   C. Blue

    B. Gray   D. Black

21. The MR image represents differences in the number of:

    A. X-rays attenuated   C. Frequencies of nuclei

    B. Nuclei and the rate of their recovery   D. Radio waves

22. The MRI process excites the nuclei in the body with:

    A. X-rays   C. Sound waves

    B. Radio waves   D. Visible light

23. The most common nuclei in the body used to receive and reemit radio waves are:

    A. Hydrogen   C. Oxygen

    B. Carbon   D. Phosphorus

24. The nuclei that receive and reemit radio waves are under the influence of:

    A. Gravitational force

    C. X-ray energy

    B. The sun and the planets

    D. A static magnetic field

25. Which of the following properties results in a nucleus behaving like a small magnet?

    A. An even number of neutrons and protons

    C. An even number of electrons

    B. An odd number of neutrons or protons

    D. The presence of a magnet

26. Precession of the magnetic nuclei occurs because of:

    A. Oscillation in the presence of other atoms

    C. The influence of a static magnetic field

    B. Regression under the influence of a magnet

    D. Ionization exposed atoms

27. A precessing nucleus produces _____ in a nearby loop of wire:

    A. An alternating current

    C. A direct current

    B. A dipole

    D. Magnetic regression

28. Precession of magnetic nuclei can be altered by the application of:

    A. X-rays

    C. Microwaves

    B. Radio frequency waves

    D. Visible light

29. Resonance occurs when radio waves are:

    A. Of the same frequency as the precessing nuclei

    C. At the same rate as T2 relaxation

    B. At the same rate as T1 relaxation

    D. Received by an antenna

30. The angle of precession of the nuclei is altered because the:

    A. Nuclei must be vertical

    C. Electrostatic properties of the nuclei dominate

    B. Magnetic force dominates

    D. MR signal is strongest when nuclei are in horizontal or transverse plane

31. Emitted signals from the exposed nuclei are _____ and sent to the computer.

    A. Evaluated

    C. In resonance

    B. Received by an RF antenna

    D. Precessing

32. The _____ among T1, T2, and spin density signals of tissues produce(s) image contrast in the MR image.

    A. Similarities

    C. Differences

    B. Phase

    D. Frequency

33. In T2 relaxation, the spins of the exposed nuclei:

    A. Are vertical in orientation

    C. Are reduced in density

    B. Move to the north

    D. Become out of phase with one another

34. In T1 relaxation, the spins of the exposed nuclei:

    A. Are relaxing back to a vertical orientation

    C. Are reduced in density

    B. Stay in a horizontal position

    D. Become out of phase with one another

35. Spin density refers to the _____ of hydrogen nuclei.

   A. Quality
   C. Phase D

   B. Quantity
   D. Wavelength

36. The signal strength and thus the brightness of points in the image are primarily determined by:

   A. Differences in T1 and T2 relaxation rates of tissues
   C. The longitudinal component of nuclei

   B. Differences in spin density of tissues
   D. Exposure of the nuclei to the static magnetic field

37. Common strengths of magnets used in MRI range from:

   A. 1 to 3 tesla
   B. 12 to 15 tesla

   B. 5 to 7 tesla
   D. 15 to 20 tesla

38. Which one of the following types of MRI magnets requires the use of cryogens?

   A. Permanent
   C. Resistive

   B. Superconducting magnets
   D. Open magnets

39. TR can be defined simply as:

   A. Time reversal
   C. Timing range

   B. Repetition time
   D. Time of resonance

40. TE can be defined simply as:

   A. Echo phase
   C. Temporary echo

   B. Time net
   D. Echo time

41. TR and TE have a profound influence on:

   A. Image noise deletion
   C. Signal averaging

   B. Image contrast
   D. Image density

42. One tesla equals:

   A. 10,000 times the earth's magnetic field
   C. 10 gauss

   B. 0.00005 gauss
   D. 10,000 gauss

43. Which one of the following is *not* a similarity between MRI and CT?

   A. The outward appearance of the unit
   C. The use of ionizing radiation

   B. The use of a computer to analyze information
   D. Images viewed as a slice of tissue

44. Primary safety concerns for the technologist, patient, and medical personnel are due to:

   A. Fringe field strengths less than 1 gauss

   B. Gravitational pull on metallic objects

   C. Magnetic fields and heat production

   D. Interaction of magnetic fields with ferrometallic objects and tissues

45. Projectiles are a concern because of:

   A. Force of ferromagnetic objects being pulled to the magnet
   C. Nerve cell function

   B. Fringe fields less than 10 gauss
   D. Local heating of tissues and metallic objects

46. Pacemakers are not allowed inside the:

    A. 5-gauss line   C. 1.0-gauss line

    B. 2.5-gauss line   D. 0.5-gauss line

47. IV pumps, wheelchairs, and O_2 tanks are not allowed inside the:

    A. 150-gauss line   C. 5-gauss line

    B. 50-gauss line   D. 1-gauss line

48. The most important MRI safety contraindication in regard to torquing of metallic objects is:

    A. Intraabdominal surgical staples   C. Ferromagnetic intracranial aneurysm clips

    B. Stainless steel femoral rods   D. Titanium hip prosthesis

49. Local heating of tissues (referred to as *SAR*, or *specific absorption ratio*) is measured in:

    A. W/kg   C. RF frequency

    B. C°   D. F°

50. The contrast agent commonly used for MR examinations is:

    A. Iodine 131   C. Gadolinium oxysulfide

    B. Lanthanum oxybromide   D. Gadolinium-diethylene triamine pentaacetic acid

51. Contrast agents are generally used in conjunction with:

    A. T1-weighted pulse sequences   C. Spin-density weighted pulse sequences

    B. T2-weighted pulse sequences   D. All of the above

52. True/False: Contrast media used in MRI carry a higher risk for reaction as compared with iodinated contrast agents.

53. Which of these pathologic indications would indicate the use of contrast media during an MRI procedure?

    A. Cerebral bleed   C. HNP

    B. C-spine fracture   D. Pituitary tumor

54. True/False: T1-weighted images will demonstrate free air within the abdominal cavity.

55. On T1-weighted images, CSF will appear:

    A. Dark   C. Same as white matter

    B. Bright   D. Same as gray matter

56. On T2-weighted images, CSF will appear:

    A. Dark   C. Same as white matter

    B. Bright   D. Same as gray matter

57. MRI of the brain allows visualization of:

    A. White matter disease   C. Small calcifications

    B. Acute cerebral bleeds   D. Skull anomalies

58. MRI of the brain includes the use of a standard head coil and:

    A. Prone position   C. Sedation

    B. Cardiac gating   D. T1- and T2-weighted pulse sequences

59. Which of the following is *not* best evaluated by MRI of the spine?

    A. Bone marrow changes   C. Disk herniation

    B. Cord abnormalities   D. Degree of scoliosis present in spine

60. MRI of the joints or limbs demonstrates all of the following *except:*

    A. Ligaments   C. Muscle

    B. Tendons   D. Cortical bone

61. The largest drawback to MRI of the abdomen is:

    A. Motion artifacts   C. Coil selection

    B. Metallic implants   D. Sequence times

62. True/False: High-field strength MRI magnets can produce up to 3 tesla.

63. 1 tesla is equal to:

    A. 1 kilogauss   C. 10,000 gauss

    B. 30,000 gauss   D. 50,000 gauss

64. A stray magnetic field that exists outside the MRI gantry is the definition for:

    A. RF field   C. Magnetic field

    B. Fringe field   D. Field of influence

65. A device for accelerating charged particles in a circular orbit to high energies by means of an alternating electric field is a:

    A. Cyclotron   C. Linear accelerator

    B. Particle accelerator   D. Pulsed accelerator

66. A helium nucleus, consisting of 2 protons and 2 neutrons, is a(n):

    A. Alpha particle   C. Beta particle

    B. Neutrino   D. Radionuclide

67. A type of atom whose nucleus disintegrates spontaneously is a(n):

    A. Alpha particle   C. Radiopharmaceutical

    B. Beta particle   D. Radionuclide

68. PET demonstrates the _____ of the body's organs and tissues.

    A. Anatomy   C. Physiology

    B. Biochemical function D. Chemical structure

69. What is produced when a positron and electron join and then undergo annihilation?

    A. X-ray   C. Radionuclide

    B. Alpha particle   D. Two 511-keV photons

70. Which of the following elements is *not* used in the PET annihilation process?

    A. Hydrogen   C. Fluorine

    B. Carbon   D. Oxygen

71. Which of the following biochemical compounds is used to gauge glucose metabolism in tissues?

    A. ^{15}O-water   C. ^{18}F-FDG

    B. ^{13}N-ammonia   D. ^{11}C-methionine

72. Most PET tracers have a half-life of:

    A. 1 to 13 seconds   C. 150 to 320 seconds

    B. 120 seconds to 110 minutes D. 8 to 12 hours

73. True/False: Malignant cells have a high rate of glucose metabolism.

74. True/False: During an epileptic seizure, there is a decrease in sugar (glucose) utilization at the seizure site in the brain.

75. Brain mapping is a PET procedure used to identify:

    A. Primary tumors   C. Critical motor or sensory regions

    B. Metastatic spread   D. Regions of brain responsible for dementia

76. True/False: CNS tumors examined with PET will demonstrate decreased glucose metabolism.

77. True/False: Dementia, when studied with PET, is demonstrated by decreased glucose metabolism in aspects of the brain.

78. The most common form of coregistration, or fusion technology is the use of:

    A. PET/MRI   C. PET/X-ray

    B. CT/MRI   D. PET/CT

79. Functional MRI is performed to study:

    A. Anatomy of the brain

    B. Specific functions of the brain

    C. Processes such as language, vision, movement, hearing, and memory

    D. All of the above

80. True/False: Functional MRI of the brain exceeds the spatial resolution seen with PET and SPECT images.

Self-Test Answers

Chapter 14
Upper Gastrointestinal System
1. C. Production of hormones
2. C. Pineal
3. Barium swallow
4. Mumps
5. A. Mastication
6. B. Epiglottis
7. D. T11
8. A. Trachea
9. Peristalsis
10. Stomach
11. D. Incisura angularis
12. A. Fundus
13. False (in the stomach)
14. False (the greater curvature)
15. Fundus
16. Head of pancreas and C-loop of duodenum
17. 1. E
    2. F
    3. I
    4. H
    5. C
    6. A
    7. D
    8. G
    9. B
18. A. Distal esophagus
    B. Region of esophagogastric junction
    C. Fundus
    D. Greater curvature
    E. Body of stomach
    F. Pylorus (pyloric antrum)
    G. Pyloric canal
    H. Pyloric orifice (sphincter)
    I. Descending portion of duodenum
    J. Duodenal bulb
    K. Lesser curvature
19. A. Prone—PA projection
    B. Air in fundus with barium in the body
20. Lateral
21. A. Supine—AP projection
    B. Barium-filled fundus (air in pylorus); also no spine rotation
22. A. Posterior—left posterior oblique position
    B. Air in pylorus with barium in the fundus indicates a semisupine position
    C. RAO
    D. Air in fundus indicates a semi-prone position and duodenal bulb and C-loop in profile indicate an RAO and not an LAO.
23. Chyme
24. A. Vitamins

25. C. Rhythmic segmentation
26. Hyposthenic or asthenic; L3-4
27. Hypersthenic, T11-12
28. Barium sulfate
29. Carbon dioxide (calcium carbonate crystals)
30. A. Three or four parts barium to one part water
    B. One part barium to one part water
31. When there is a possibility that the contrast media may spill into the peritoneum (such as presurgery or a perforated bowel)
32. C. Dehydration
33. A. True
34. Output
35. C. 1000 to 6000 times
36. True
37. Lower
38. Distance
39. B. 0.50 mm Pb/Eq.
40. A. Zenker's diverticulum
41. A. Esophageal reflux
42. D. Antral muscle thickness exceeding 4 mm
43. B. Nuclear medicine
44. D. Trapped vegetable fiber in the stomach
45. To detect signs of esophageal reflux (GERD)
46. 35° to 40°
47. The RAO places the esophagus between the heart and vertebra better than an LAO.
48. Majority of esophagus is superimposed over the spine and thus is not well visualized
49. Shredded cotton or marshmallows
50. Right lateral position
51. Reduce patient rotation to less than 40 degrees for an asthenic patient.
52. AP projection performed recumbent
53. To rule out esophageal varices (a condition of dilation of the veins, which in advanced stages may lead to internal bleeding)
54. The Valsalva maneuver, to rule out esophageal reflux (a condition wherein gastric contents return back through the gastric orifice into the esophagus, causing irritation of esophageal lining)
55. An ulcer
56. A. 125 kV
57. Left posterior oblique (LPO) recumbent
58. B. Bucky slot shield
59. Sliding hiatal hernia

60. A mass of hair trapped in the stomach. An upper GI study may be performed to diagnose this condition.

Chapter 15
Lower Gastrointestinal System
1. A. 15 to 18 ft (4.5 to 5.5 m)
2. C. Ileum
3. D. Suspensory ligament of the duodenum
4. A. Ileum
5. C. Jejunum
6. A. Cecum
   B. Rectum
7. Vermiform appendix
8. True
9. False (in large intestine)
10. Left
11. A. Jejunum
    B. Ileum
    C. Region of ileocecal sphincter (valve)
    D. Duodenum (C-loop)
    E. Pyloric portion of stomach
    F. Left colic (splenic) flexure
    G. Descending colon
    H. Sigmoid colon
    I. Rectum
    J. Cecum
    K. Ascending colon
    L. Right colic (hepatic) flexure
    M. Transverse colon
12. C. Transverse colon
13. B. Large intestine
14. B. Rhythmic segmentation
15. 1. F
    2. D
    3. I
    4. L
    5. B
    6. G
    7. J
    8. C
    9. A
    10. E
    11. M
    12. K
    13. H
16. 1. D
    2. G
    3. E
    4. H
    5. A
    6. C
    7. B
    8. F
17. A. Barium enema
18. False

19. Hold breath on expiration
20. Produces compression of the abdomen that leads to separation of the loops of small intestine
21. 8 hours
22. Cathartic
23. Rectal retention enema tip
24. Glucagon
25. Lidocaine
26. D. Prolapse of rectum
27. B. Anorectal angle
28. True
29. RAO position
30. 2 hours
31. D. Anatrast
32. C. Center chamber only
33. 35° to 45°
34. 2 inches (5 cm)
35. Defecography
36. LPO position
37. Right lateral decubitus will drain excess barium from the descending colon allowing for detection of small polyps
38. Evacuative proctography
39. False
40. False
41. True
42. D. 2000 to 3000 mrad
43. A. Right; iliac crest
    B. Left; 1 to 2 inches (2.5 to 5 cm) above the iliac crest
44. False
45. A. RPO
46. C. Enteroclysis
47. Nuclear medicine
48. A. Wear gloves
49. Sprue
50. True

Chapter 16
Gallbladder and Biliary Ducts
1. A. Anterior inferior
2. C. Inferior
3. D. Right upper quadrant
4. Falciform ligament
5. To break down or emulsify fats
6. Common hepatic duct
7. 30 to 40 ml
8. Hydrolysis
9. Cholecystokinin (CCK)
10. Common bile duct (CBD)
11. 1. H
    2. F
    3. G
    4. A
    5. I
    6. B
    7. D
    8. E
    9. C

12. A. Supine
    B. Because the body and fundus of the gallbladder are anterior and the neck and cystic duct are posterior
13. A. Fundus
    B. Body
    C. Neck
    D. Cystic duct
    E. Duodenum
    F. Common bile duct
    G. Common hepatic duct
    H. Right hepatic duct
    I. Left hepatic duct
14. 1. H
    2. I
    3. A
    4. B
    5. C
    6. F
    7. E
    8. G
    9. D
15. False
16. True
17. 1. C
    2. D
    3. E
    4. G
    5. B
    6. A
    7. F
18. At least 8 hours
19. 10 to 12 hours before the procedure (minimum)
20. 70 to 76 kV
21. False (the patient needs to be NPO only 4 hours before the ultrasound procedure)
22. True
23. Through a special catheter introduced through the duodenoscope
24. B. Pneumothorax
25. Endoscopic retrograde cholangiopancreatography
26. Gastroenterologist
27. To detect postoperatively any residual stones in the biliary ducts that may have gone undetected during the cholecystectomy
28. B. Obstructive jaundice
29. D. Skinny, or Chiba, needle
30. A. R
    B. S
    C. R
31. True
32. True
33. True
34. False
35. True
36. Center chamber

37. Low, approximately the level of the iliac crest and near the midline of the body
38. Increase the rotation of the body for the LAO position.
39. Because of the more anterior location of the gallbladder producing less magnification of it
40. Either the erect PA projection or a right lateral decubitus position will stratify or "layer" any possible stones in the gallbladder.
41. RPO position
42. Keep the patient NPO for 4 hours; then perform a sonographic study of the gallbladder.
43. B. CT of the gallbladder

Chapter 17
Urinary System
1. A. Retroperitoneal
2. C. Posterolateral
3. Anterior
4. 30°
5. A. Ureteropelvic junction (UPJ)
   B. Near brim of pelvis
   C. Ureterovesical junction (UVJ)
6. 2 inches; 5 cm
7. Uremia
8. D. 1.5 liters
9. D. Inferior vena cava
10. Renal pyramids
11. Renal pelvis
12. Nephron
13. True
14. False (99% is reabsorbed.)
15. Trigone
16. A. Urinary bladder
    B. Midureter
    C. Ureteropelvic junction (UPJ)
    D. Renal pelvis
    E. Major calyces
    F. Minor calyces
17. Retrograde pyelogram (note catheter in right ureter)
18. When the benefit of the procedure outweighs the risks of the radiation exposure
19. Ionic and nonionic
20. A. I
    B. N
    C. I
    D. I
    E. I
    F. N
    G. I
    H. N
    I. I
    J. N

21. B. 0.6 to 1.5 mg/dl
22. A. 48 hours
23. B. Pheochromocytoma
24. A. Observe and reassure patient
25. A. Vasomotor effect
26. C. Anaphylactic reaction
27. C. Anaphylactic
28. B. Vasovagal reaction
29. D. Lasix
30. B. Diabetes
31. A. Prednisone
32. C. Oliguria
33. D. Urinary incontinence
34. A. Renal agenesis
35. B. Anuria
36. True
37. A. Renal cell carcinoma
38. B. Mild level reaction
39. D. Severe level reaction
40. A. Side effect
41. C. Axillary
42. 20° to 45°
43. Anuria, or anuresis
44. Lithotripsy
45. D. Vesicourethral reflux
46. A. Renal obstruction
47. A. Ectopic kidney
48. True
49. True
50. B. Ureteric calculi
51. 20 minutes following injection
52. Nephrogram or nephrotomography; immediately after completion of injection
53. Retrograde urethrogram on a male patient
54. Left posterior oblique (LPO)
55. False (higher for female)
56. False (primarily the ureter)
57. Angle the CR more caudally to project the symphysis pubis inferior to the bladder.
58. 30 seconds to 1 minute following the start of the bolus injection
59. Place the patient in a 15° Trendelenburg position during first aspect of procedure.
60. Overrotation of the body will foreshorten the kidney and superimpose it over the spine.

Chapter 18
Mammography

1. Mammography Quality Standards Act; 1994
2. Only Veterans Administration (VA) facilities
3. 40
4. 8
5. Inframammary crease
6. Upper outer quadrant (UOQ)
7. 11 o'clock
8. Pectoralis major muscle
9. Lactation, or production of milk
10. Cooper's ligaments
11. Adipose (fatty)
12. Trabeculae
13. Base
14. A. Fibro-glandular
15. B. Fibro-fatty
16. C. Fatty
17. A. Fibro-fatty
18. A. Glandular tissue
    B. Nipple
    C. Adipose (fatty) tissue
    D. Pectoral muscle
    E. Mediolateral oblique (MLO)
    F. Axillary
19. Molybdenum
20. Apex
21. True (only time it cannot be used is with implants)
22. True
23. False (Grid is used because of the large amount of scatter and secondary radiation.)
24. 0.1 mm
25. 2 times the original size of the object
26. B. 200 to 300 mrad (130 to 150 per projection)
27. Sonography (ultrasound)
28. Magnetic resonance imaging (MRI)
29. True
30. False (Patient dose is reduced primarily by minimizing repeats.)
31. True
32. A. Sulfur colloid
33. Noninvasive and invasive
34. D. XCCL
35. MLO
36. A. Craniocaudal (CC)
    B. Mediolateral oblique (MLO)
37. Mediolateral oblique projection
38. 25 to 28 kV
39. Exaggerated craniocaudal–lateral (XCCL) projection
40. LMO
41. Overexposure
42. A. Eklund
    B. Implant-displaced (ID)
43. Axillary tail view (AT)
44. Axillary side
45. Have patient hold the breast back with her opposite hand.
46. MLO (mediolateral oblique)
47. XCCL (exaggerated craniocaudad–lateral)
48. Inframammary crease at its upper limits
49. B. Mediolateral oblique
50. C. Use manual exposure factors
51. D. Flat panel receptor
52. False
53. Computer-aided detection
54. 10%

55. A. Technetium-99m-sestamibi
56. Metabolism
57. False
58. C. MRI
59. B. High false-positive rate
60. D. Infiltrating ductal carcinoma

Chapter 19
Trauma, Mobile, and Surgical Radiography

1. A. Spiral fracture
   B. Compound fracture
   C. Comminuted fracture
   D. Greenstick fracture
   E. Colles' fracture
   F. Impacted fracture
   G. Compression fracture
   H. Stellate fracture
   I. Pott's fracture
2. A. Dislocation or luxation
   B. Subluxation
3. Spine (although it can occur in the elbow as well)
4. B. Lack of apposition
5. A. Valgus angulation
6. A. 5
   B. 9
   C. 4
   D. 8
   E. 1
   F. 2
   G. 3
   H. 7
   I. 6
7. True
8. True
9. D. AP shoulder
10. B. 6:1 to 8:1
11. A. Grid frequency
    B. Grid ratio
12. True
13. Battery-operated, battery-driven
14. Standard power source
15. False (mobile fluoroscopy units)
16. True
17. False (PA is recommended because of less exposure to operator and less OID.)
18. True
19. Road-mapping
20. Reducing patient dose
21. A. Time
    B. Distance
    C. Shielding
22. Distance
23. A. Less than 10 mR/hr
24. 4 mR ($30 \div 60 \times 8 = 4$)
25. False (greater on tube side)
26. False (by a factor of 4)
27. A. Right lateral decubitus
28. 3 to 4 inches (7 to 10 cm) below the jugular notch

29. 15° to 20° mediolateral angle and horizontal beam lateral projections
30. C. Left lateral decubitus
31. Two
32. Parallel to the interepicondylar plane
33. A horizontal beam lateromedial projection
34. 25° to 30°, or until the CR can be projected parallel to the scapular blade (wing)
35. 10° posteriorly from perpendicular to the plantar surface of the foot
36. Perform a cross-angle CR projection of the ankle, with CR 15° to 20° lateromedial from the long axis of the foot.
37. C. The affected leg is rotated 10° to 20° internally if possible
38. A. 35° to 40° cephalad AP axial projection
39. C. Perform a double-angle oblique with IR perpendicular to CR
40. A. It reduces distortion
    B. The long OID produces an air gap effect, which improves image quality without the use of a grid, thus allowing a double CR angle (which would cause grid cutoff if a grid were used).
41. B. Trauma, horizontal beam lateral
42. A. Crosswise
    B. 2 inches (5 cm) superior to EAM
43. C. Lateral
44. A. AP or PA and lateral wrist
45. D. Epiphyseal
46. B. Trauma axiolateral projection
47. D. Anesthesiologist
48. Certified surgical technologist
49. C. Surgical assistant
50. A. Shower curtain
51. C. Asepsis
52. A. Only the level of the tabletop
53. False
54. True
55. True
56. D. Weekly
57. C. Use intermittent fluoroscopy
58. A. Shallow RPO
59. True
60. Nonfunctional
61. Pelvicalyceal
62. Open reduction with internal fixation
63. B. Intramedullary rod
64. D. Ilizarov device
65. D. All of the above require fluoroscopic guidance
66. D. Interbody fusion cage
67. A. Scoliosis corrective surgery
68. Kirschner wires
69. Fracture or orthopedic table
70. Dynamic hip screw

Chapter 20
Pediatric Radiography

1. B. 2 years
2. D. Describe the total amount of radiation the patient will receive with that specific exam if it has to be repeated because of a lack of cooperation
3. D. Do none of the above
4. D. Hold-em Tiger
5. C. Pigg-O-Stat
6. A. Proper immobilization
   B. Short exposure times
   C. Accurate technique charts
7. Are you pregnant?
8. C. Pigg-O-Stat
9. D. 3-D ultrasound
10. B. Functional MRI
11. A. 4
    B. 9
    C. 7
    D. 2
    E. 13
    F. 3
    G. 12
    H. 11
    I. 1
    J. 6
    K. 10
    L. 8
    M. 5
12. A. (+)
    B. (+)
    C. (−)
    D. (+)
    E. (−)
    F. (+)
    G. (−)
13. C. Extend arms upward
14. 55 to 65 kV
15. True
16. True
17. Kite method
18. Between the umbilicus and just above the pubis
19. 1. D
    2. E
    3. EP
    4. D
    5. E and EP
20. A. 2
    B. 2
    C. 5
    D. 1
    E. 5
    F. 4
    G. 1
    H. 2
    I. 4
    J. 1
    K. 5
    L. 1
    M. 1
21. D. 30°

22. B. Midway between glabella and inion
23. A. 4 hours
24. Diminish the risk for aspiration from vomiting
25. C. Appendicitis
26. A. Level of iliac crest
    B. 1 inch (2.5 cm) above umbilicus
27. Mammillary (nipple) level
28. 6 to 12 ounces
29. Manually, very slowly, using a 60-ml syringe and a #10 French flexible silicone catheter
30. No bowel prep is required.
31. When the bladder is full and when voiding
32. 1
33. A. Vesicoureteral reflux
    B. Before
34. False (Shielding should be used in all positions, using tape when necessary.)
35. True
36. B. AP and lateral upper airway
37. D. AP and lateral knee
38. B. Inform supervisor or physician
39. C. Spina bifida
40. D. Functional MRI (fMRI)

Chapter 21
Angiography and Interventional Procedures

1. D. Right and left coronary arteries
2. D. Right common carotid
3. A. C4 vertebra
4. A. Pulmonary veins
5. C. Right common carotid
6. A. Anterior portion of brain
7. B. Anterior and middle cerebral arteries
8. D. Basilar artery
9. D. Sphenoid
10. C. Internal and external cerebral veins
11. B. Internal jugular vein
12. C. Azygos vein
13. 1. E
    2. J
    3. D
    4. I
    5. K
    6. B
    7. F
    8. H
    9. G
    10. A
    11. L
    12. C
14. False (from brachiocephalic artery)
15. False (median cubital vein)
16. True
17. True
18. C. Aortic root
19. B. Four

20. B. Inverse aorta
21. A. Portal vein
22. B. Synthesize simple carbohydrates
23. C. 8
24. C. Femoral artery
25. 1. O
    2. Q
    3. P
    4. N
    5. L
    6. D
    7. A
    8. K
    9. R
    10. M
    11. G
    12. C
    13. F
    14. B
    15. H
26. C. Body temperature
27. B. Color duplex ultrasound
28. B. 4 hours
29. D. Flat detector fluoroscopy
30. False
31. True
32. False (does not need to be used)
33. True
34. C. Coarctation
35. C. 8 to 10 seconds
36. B. Pulmonary emboli
37. A. Femoral vein
38. C. 45° LAO
39. C. Left ventricle
40. D. 15 to 30 frames per second
41. D. Bowel obstruction
42. C. 30 to 40 ml
43. True
44. A. Helps to visualize the lymph vessels
45. True
46. False (Oil-based is used. Water-soluble is too quickly absorbed.)
47. D. Malignancies
48. A. 3
    B. 4
    C. 6
    D. 1
    E. 7
    F. 2
    G. 5
49. False (placed inferior to renal veins)
50. True

Chapter 22
Computed Tomography

1. A. First generation
2. C and D. Third- and fourth-generation
3. Slip rings
4. A. 1%
5. Postpatient collimator
6. Assign various shades of gray to the CT numbers

7. A. Gantry
   B. Computer
   C. Operator console
8. Pixel
9. D. Vertical adjustment of table height
10. B. Voxel
11. True
12. D. 40
13. Attenuation
14. Water
15. Zero (0)
16. A. –100
17. C. Slice thickness
18. B. 2:1
19. True
20. Blood-brain
21. C. Multiple sclerosis
22. B and E. Possible neoplasia and brain tumor
23. A. Dendrites
    B. Axon
24. Meninges
25. A. Dura mater
    B. Arachnoid mater
    C. Pia mater
26. A. Pia mater
    B. Arachnoid mater
    C. Dura mater
    D. Venous sinus
    E. Epidural space
    F. Subdural space
    G. Subarachnoid spaces
27. Subarachnoid space
28. A. 3
    B. 3
    C. 1
    D. 1
    E. 3
29. Cerebrum
30. Longitudinal fissure
31. Corpus callosum
32. Falx cerebri
33. A. Lateral ventricles
34. C. Cisterna cerebellomedullaris
35. A. Lateral
    B. Third
    C. Fourth
       a. Interventricular foramen
       b. Cerebral aqueduct
       c. Lateral recess
          1. Body
          2. Anterior horn
          3. Inferior (temporal) horn
          4. Posterior horn
          5. Pineal gland
36. Hydrocephalus; ventricles
37. Cisterns
38. A. Frontal
    B. Parietal
    C. Occipital
    D. Temporal
    E. Insula or central lobe

39. A. 1
    B. 2
    C. 2
    D. 1
    E. 2
    F. 1
40. B. Inferior portion of manubrium
41. A. Sternal notch
42. C. Aortopulmonary window
43. A. Base of heart
44. Aortopulmonary window
45. A. Ascending aorta
46. C. Left atrium
47. D. Mitral valve prolapse
48. A. 10 mm
49. D. The hook-like extension of the head of the pancreas
50. D. All of the above
51. D. All of the above
52. D. Symphysis pubis
53. C. Urinary bladder
54. B. 10 mm
55. D. Answers A and C
56. C. Xiphoid process
57. True
58. False (They speed up peristaltic action.)
59. False (Patients need to hold breath.)
60. True
61. True
62. C. 20 seconds
63. A. 3 to 5 mm
64. C. Air
65. True
66. Multiplanar reconstruction (MPR)
67. Window width

Chapter 23
Additional Diagnostic Procedures

1. Orthoroentgenography
2. False (Ends of bone must be on separate projections.)
3. False (a premature fusion of the epiphysis to shorten a bone)
4. True
5. True
6. Bell-Thompson ruler
7. 24 × 39 cm (10 × 12 inches) or 30 × 35 cm (11 × 14 inches) with three exposures placed on the same IR
8. A. Knee
   B. Shoulder
9. A. Sensitivity to iodine
   B. Sensitivity to local anesthetics
10. Knee
11. A. Iodinated water soluble, approximately 5 ml
    B. Carbon dioxide, oxygen or room air, 80 to 100 ml
12. 20 gauge
13. To provide a thin, even coating of positive contrast media over the soft tissues of the knee joint

14. 35 × 43 cm (14 × 17 inches) or 18 × 43 cm (7 × 17 inches)
15. A. 6
    B. 30°
16. The conjoined tendons of the four major shoulder muscles
17. Spinal needle
18. A. AP internal and external rotation shoulder scout
    B. AP internal rotation
    C. AP external rotation
    D. Glenoid fossa projection (Grashey method)
    E. Transaxillary (inferosuperior axial) projection
    F. Bicipital (intertubercular) groove projection (Fisk method)
19. A. Herniated nucleus pulposus (HNP)
    B. Cancerous or benign tumors
    C. Cysts
    D. Possible bone fragments (trauma)
20. A. Blood in the cerebrospinal fluid
    B. Arachnoiditis
    C. Increased intracranial pressure
    D. Recent lumbar puncture (within the past 2 weeks)
21. C. HNP
22. Subarachnoid space
23. C. Trendelenburg
24. A. L3-4
25. D. The patient has complete blockage at T-spine level
26. 30 minutes; 24 hours
27. Horizontal beam swimmer's lateral
28. Body section radiography
29. A. 4
    B. 6
    C. 3
    D. 1
    E. 5
    F. 2
30. True
31. False (is the exposure angle)
32. True
33. False
34. True
35. True
36. A. 2 to 3 seconds
37. A. Fundus
    B. Corpus or body
    C. Isthmus
    D. Cervix (neck)
38. A. Osseometrium
39. False (connected to the uterus at the corna)
40. A. Acute pelvic inflammatory disease
    B. Active uterine bleeding
    C. Pregnancy
41. False (Water-soluble is preferred.)
42. True
43. A. 2
    B. 3

C. 1
44. B. Severe inflammation of the salivary gland or duct
45. Water-soluble contrast media
46. Dilation of the salivary duct
47. A. Excessive physical activity
48. A. Fan-beam x-ray source
49. B. Young healthy individual with peak bone mass
50. A. Higher patient dose
    B. More expensive as compared with other bone densitometry systems
51. Os calcis or calcaneus
52. Osteoclasts
53. C. Undergoing glucocorticoid therapy
54. False
55. B. Osteopenia
56. False
57. A. 1 to 30 μSv
58. True
59. C. L1 to L4
60. Precision (or reproducibility)

Chapter 24
Additional Diagnostic and Therapeutic Modalities

1. B. Technetium 99m
2. A. SPECT camera
3. B. Hot spot
4. C. Meckel's diverticulum
5. D. Vasodilator
6. False (during the ventilation phase)
7. A. Calibrates instrumentation
8. B. Neutron accelerator
9. D. 4 to 30 MeV
10. True
11. C. Prescribes the treatment
12. C. Piezosonography
13. D. 1 to 17 MHz
14. B. B-mode
15. A. Electrical
16. A. 3.5 MHz
17. False (decreased penetration but higher resolution)
18. False (Gallbladder is anechoic.)
19. True
20. C. Blue
21. B. Nuclei and the rate of their recovery
22. B. Radio waves
23. A. Hydrogen
24. D. A static magnetic field
25. B. An odd number of neutrons or protons
26. C. The influence of a static magnetic field
27. A. An alternating current
28. B. Radio frequency waves
29. A. Of the same frequency as the precessing nuclei
30. D. MR signal is strongest when nuclei are in horizontal or transverse plane

31. B. Received by an RF antenna
32. C. Differences
33. D. Become out of phase with one another
34. A. Are relaxing back to a vertical orientation (within the magnetic field)
35. B. Quantity
36. A. Differences in T1 and T2 relaxation rates of tissues nuclei
37. A. 1 to 3 tesla
38. B. Superconducting magnets
39. B. Repetition time
40. D. Echo time
41. B. Image contrast
42. D. 10,000 gauss
43. C. The use of ionizing radiation
44. D. Interaction of magnetic fields with ferrometallic objects and tissues
45. A. Force of ferrometallic objects being pulled to the magnet
46. A. 5-gauss line
47. B. 50-gauss line
48. C. Ferromagnetic intracranial aneurysm clips
49. A. W/kg
50. D. Gadolinium-diethylene triamine pentaacetic acid
51. A. T1-weighted pulse sequences
52. False
53. D. Pituitary tumor
54. False
55. A. Dark
56. B. Bright
57. A. White matter disease
58. D. T1- and T2-weighted pulse sequences
59. D. Degree of scoliosis present in spine
60. D. Cortical bone
61. A. Motion artifacts
62. True
63. C. 10,000 gauss
64. B. Fringe field
65. A. Cyclotron
66. A. Alpha particle
67. D. Radionuclide
68. B. Biochemical function
69. D. Two 511-keV photons
70. A. Hydrogen
71. C. ^{18}F-FDG
72. B. 120 seconds to 110 minutes
73. True
74. False
75. C. Critical motor or sensory regions
76. False
77. True
78. D. PET/CT
79. D. All of the above
80. True